DRIFT

LIFE'S FRACTURED FOUNDATION

WAYNE WATTERS

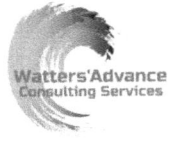

Watters'Advance
Consulting Services

CHAPTER 1
PATTERNS IN THE NOISE

Micah Vasquez is six years old, bright-eyed and small for his age, with an easy laugh that charms even the older kids. He likes dinosaurs and string cheese, and on most days, recess is his favorite part of school. Today, though, something feels off.

Micah's fingers curl tightly around the rusting chain of the swing, feet dragging shallow channels in the mulch. Around him, children shout, run, and kick up dust in the air. It's warm. Warmer than expected, according to his mom. Micah is more aware of how bright it is. There's no cloud in the sky.

He stays still, letting the swing sway with the breeze that carries a sharp scent of the nearby dumpsters. His eyes follow a boy in a green shirt climbing the wall of tires, then his attention is pulled to the basketball court, where someone whistles and laughter erupts. He wants to join them and feel his shoes slap the pavement, but something in his chest pulls at him, and he stays put. It feels like a quiet warning he can't make sense of. His legs feel heavy, the way they do when he runs too hard during tag, only he hasn't moved. Just five more minutes, he tells himself, then I'll go. But even that feels like a promise he's not sure he can keep.

He doesn't know why he feels so heavy. Like the air has grown thick. Like his thoughts are trying to swim through syrup. A soft sound hums at the edges of his hearing, like someone breathing through a cracked door. He blinks hard.

Then everything slows.

The sunlight bends around his vision, casting halos around the moving shapes. The other children blur like echoes of themselves; their motions become too fast and too slow all at once. A strange pressure builds behind his eyes, as if something is folding inward. His hands tremble, one slipping from the chain. He tries to call out, to say his teacher's name, but his tongue feels swollen, detached, as though his voice has been packed in cotton. Sound dulls, then rings sharply. Every noise is both distant and too close, like a balloon popping inside his skull. The mulch under his shoes pulses as if it were breathing. Then it vanishes into an overwhelming burst of light and stars.

He falls sideways off the swing, unable to control the fall and unsure which way is up. He feels the impact of hitting the ground as everything goes dark.

Teachers come running. Someone screams. Micah's body twists in the mulch, muscles seizing, eyes wide and vacant. For three long minutes, the schoolyard freezes in collective fear.

Ms. Noelle is the first to act. She's the first-grade teacher every child wishes they had, with her bright purple hair and often playing video games with the kids after school while waiting for parents to arrive. Noelle quickly reaches Micah and drops to her knees beside him, trying to steady his flailing limbs with shaking hands. "It's probably heat exhaustion," someone mutters, though it's not hot enough for that.

Another teacher, Ms. Jazmin, runs for water, yelling for the nurse and for someone to call 9 1 1 as she goes.

The P.E. coach, Mr. Jason, known for driving a truck so big that it requires two parking spots, opens his jacket and stretches it overhead to cast shade across Micah's body. Jason's eyes scan Micah's face for any sign that he can hear him.

"Micah, my man, can you hear me? You're okay, you're safe," he proclaims, his voice trembling. But nothing about this feels okay. Micah's jaw is locked, and his fists are clenched. A trail of drool shines in the mulch beneath his cheek.

The children are all hustled back as Nurse Peter is seen coming in. They cluster near the school doors, some are crying, while others are just staring. The world has gone quiet, except for the sound of Jason's voice repeating Micah's name like a prayer against the chaos.

The school nurse arrives in a sprint. As Peter approaches, Jason quickly steps aside to give him room, still holding the jacket aloft to shield Micah from the sun. Peter kneels down, focused and efficient. "Micah," he proclaims. "We've called your mom. She's on her way."

Peter's a tall, thin man, standing six feet five inches tall with thick brown hair and blue eyes. As a young adult, he had difficulty communicating with kids, but they gravitated to him just the same. Outsiders mistook the awkward communication as indifference, but his empathy and nurturing nature make him uniquely skilled for medical care. Peter arrives on the scene, racing into action.

Peter drops to his knees beside Micah, quickly assessing Micah's airway, breathing, and circulation. Micah is breathing irregularly. His pulse is fast. Peter gently rolls him to his side into the recovery position, placing a folded gym mat under Micah's head to prevent injury.

He notes the clenched jaw, the tremors still pulsing through Micah's limbs, and the fine mist of sweat over his brow. "Let him ride it out," Peter says. "Don't try to hold him still. We just keep him safe."

Still kneeling beside Micah, Noelle swallows hard and nods, trying to steady her breath. "Okay, just keep him safe," she repeats quietly, her voice barely audible. Then, glancing at Peter, she asks, "How long do we wait?"

Reaching into his kit, Peter pulls out a stopwatch and begins timing. The seizure was already past the one-minute mark. "If he doesn't start to come out in another minute, we'll prep the emergency meds."

He speaks calmly, but his mind races through protocols, trying to remember his training.

When the seizure finally subsides, Micah lies still. Peter places a hand gently on the boy's shoulder. His stopwatch reads forty-five seconds since he started it, though it feels much longer. Relief flickers across his face as he exhales. He thinks to himself how grateful he is that they didn't have to administer the emergency meds, grateful that Micah was able to climb out of it on his own. "Micah, can you hear me, buddy? You're okay. You're safe now."

But Micah doesn't respond.

Peter waves a hand lightly in front of his face, then leans in close, checking his pupils. "Still nonresponsive," he mutters. He taps lightly on Micah's collarbone, then tries calling his name more firmly this time. "Micah. It's Peter. You're safe. Can you squeeze my hand?"

Nothing.

Behind him, shoes run through the gravel and into the mulch. A woman's voice calls out, sharp with panic: "Micah!"

Lena runs across the playground, breathless. Lena is the counselor on campus, helping students develop social skills, manage emotions, and build resilience. Right now, her eyes are locked on her son. "Is he okay? What happened? Oh my God, is he breathing?"

Peter stands, intercepting her gently with both hands raised. "He's breathing. His vitals are stable, but he's coming out of the seizure. He's just not fully aware yet."

Lena drops to her knees beside Micah, brushing the hair from his damp forehead. "Sweetheart, I'm here. I'm right here."

Peter gives her a moment, then nods toward the approaching stretcher. "The paramedics are here. They're going to take him to the hospital now. They'll get answers. I promise you, we're doing everything right."

Then they both look up at the approaching paramedics.

Andrew Turbin pulls up a dataset on his tablet in a small conference room at Dell Children's Medical Center three miles away. Andrew is a renowned doctor who is sympathetic to his patients while fumbling with emotions in his personal life. Andrew turns the screen of his tablet toward his colleague, Dr. Theo Manning. Theo is a mop-haired molecular biologist with the energy of a graduate student and the brain of a chess master.

"You're telling me this is new?" Theo asks, arms crossed.

Andrew offers a dry laugh. "I'm telling you it's accelerating. Look at autism spectrum disorder. Back in 1970, it was estimated that there were fewer than one in 10,000 children. By 1985, that jumped to one in twenty-five hundred. Then one in 150 by the turn of the century."

He pauses, turning the tablet so Theo can see the rising line on a graph. "Today, the CDC estimates one in thirty-six. And before you say it, it's not just better awareness or improved screening. The models that adjust for that still show a dramatic rise."

Theo stares at the numbers. "That looks like a measurable climb over a single generation."

"Exactly, and autism's just the start." Andrew taps again and brings up a new graph. "Congenital heart defects. In the 1970s, we saw them in about one in 1,200 newborns. Now it's one in a hundred. That's a massive shift."

Theo blinks in surprise while absorbing the information. "I thought that rate only jumped in certain regions."

"True, but now it's global," Andrew offers. "Urban centers are hit harder, but rural areas aren't immune. And that's not even accounting for underreporting in low-income regions."

Andrew flips to another chart. "Neural tube defects like spina bifida and anencephaly are up sixty-two percent since 1995. Even with folic acid widely available."

"I thought folic acid was supposed to improve that."

"It was. It is," Andrew interrupts. "But it's not enough, and we don't know why."

Andrew swiped again. "Cerebral palsy. Limb reduction anomalies. They're all trending upward. ADHD used to be five percent; now it's pushing thirteen percent in some studies. That's more than one in ten kids."

Theo lets out a low whistle. "This isn't one condition. It's a whole ecosystem shifting."

"Exactly. It's not just autism. It's everywhere. Across systems. Across countries. And across disciplines. It's not confined to one specialty's territory. Neurologists are seeing unexplained spikes in seizure disorders. Cardiologists are tracking surges in congenital defects that defy known risk factors. Developmental pediatricians are reporting higher rates of language and learning delays. Even specialists in orthopedics and craniofacial surgery are noticing subtle trends in anomalies that were once considered rare. It's as if every field that treats children is logging a separate chapter of the same story, but no one's stitched those chapters the yet to see the whole picture."

Theo shakes his head. "Pollution, pesticides, and genetics. It all makes sense. At least it adds up on paper. That's where most people stop looking."

"It is," Andrew says, softer now. "But the tangle's growing. Childhood epilepsy has more than doubled. Rare chromosome deletions are no longer rare. Even speech disorders are up to one in twelve children now. They all carry the same signatures with elevated rates, unclear causes, and rising complexity." He looks back at Theo. "The data tells a story, and we're not listening hard enough."

Theo frowns. "Why aren't we?" he asks. The question lands heavier than either expects. Andrew rubs his temple, letting the silence stretch.

"Part of it is silos," Andrew says finally. "Each specialty guards its data, publishes within its lane, and rarely connects findings across disciplines. Neurologists talk to neurologists, geneticists talk to geneticists. Nobody's stepping far enough back to see the pattern emerge."

He pauses and flips the tablet back to the first chart. "And part of it is expectation bias. We've been conditioned to think some level of increase is normal due to pollution, environmental stressors, and modern diets. When a new study confirms what people already suspect, it feels like old news instead of alarm bells. So, we categorize it as expected rather than exceptional."

Theo nods, his expression tightening. "So the rise hides in plain sight."

"Exactly," Andrew says. "Each field normalizes the slope within its own context. When looked at separately, a ten percent rise in cardiology or a twenty percent rise in developmental pediatrics looks manageable. But together, they form an exponential curve that no one charts. And then there's funding. The grants go to narrowly defined projects, not broad correlation studies. Everyone's chasing the same piece instead of assembling the puzzle."

He looks up again, his voice low but steady. "We're not ignoring it out of indifference. We're drowning in noise. But if we don't start connecting these signals soon, the next generation of data will make this look like the calm before the storm."

Before Theo can respond, Andrew's pager vibrates against the table. He glances down. "Cho needs a consult," he says. "Pediatric intake. A child was brought in from a school playground. Seizure."

Theo starts to say something, but Andrew is already on his feet, sliding the tablet into his bag. The conversation's weight follows him out the door, its unanswered questions echoing beneath the fluorescent hum of the hallway. He knows the statistics are abstract until they have a face.

By the time he reaches the elevator, Andrew is shifting into clinician mode. The data fades to the background, replaced by the practical rhythm of triage. Still, Theo's words linger in his mind: So, the rise hides in plain sight. The elevator doors close, sealing the thought inside with him as he rides toward the pediatric wing where Micah Vasquez is being prepared for intake.

CHAPTER 2
SILENCE BETWEEN BEATS

The EEG monitor beeps in a steady rhythm. Just another pulse in the ICU's mechanical symphony. Andrew Turbin sits beside Micah Vasquez, a frail-looking boy with olive skin and a soft curl of hair over one eye. Having collapsed during recess, some of the teachers at Angelina Eberly Elementary School assume heat exhaustion, but the ambulance crew arrives to find him unresponsive and deep in a seizure. Andrew reads Micah's chart and sees that after arriving at the hospital, Micah's initial scan reveals diffuse cortical irritation, with no clear cause.

Now, as sedation wears off, Micah's brain activity returns to a manageable rhythm, but Andrew remains uneasy. It's not the numbers; they are trending clean. Micah demonstrates the kind of textbook rebound that looks comforting on a chart yet collides with a strange static in Andrew's gut. It's a low, prickling signal that something more is unfolding beneath the surface. In Andrew's eyes, Micah looks fragile, his eyelids fluttering as if chasing some dream just out of reach, a faint crease between his brows hinting at effort or confusion even in sleep.

Andrew stands with Dr. Rebekah Cho, near Micah's bed, as the monitors hum softly.

"First seizure?" he asks quietly, aware that Micah's mother is asleep in the chair next to Micah's bed. Andrew follows the family-first approach when discussing the case at the bedside, even if a parent is sleeping nearby. If the parent is exhausted and the patient is stable, it's common courtesy to let them rest while the physicians quietly review the case.

Rebekah frowns and scrolls through her tablet. She nods, saying, "First and violent. No clear trigger, no family history. Birth was normal. Developmental milestones all clean. Every test comes back textbook."

Andrew asks, searching for answers, "Was there head trauma? Stroke? Infection?"

Rebekah answers flatly, "Nothing. Labs are clean. Blood sugar and sodium are steady, and metabolic panels are unremarkable. He's as balanced as a case study could be. His brain isn't reacting to an electrolyte imbalance, and chemical markers show no hint of a hidden metabolic disorder."

Andrew glances toward Micah, whose small chest rises and falls under the blanket. "Except for the part where his brain decided to short-circuit."

Rebekah continues reading from her tablet, "According to the intake, there has been no recent illness, no high fever, and no indication that Micah has experienced prolonged sleep disruption or severe psychological stress."

Andrew turns toward her, "Everything the textbooks tell us to rule out has been ruled out. Sometimes the brain misfires without warning. No damage, no injury, no infection. Just a blank space in the middle of the story."

Rebekah exhales, shaking her head. "Idiopathic," she repeats quietly. "The word we use when we run out of answers." She glances at her tablet, then looks toward the hall. "I need to sign out a patient being released. Do you have it covered?"

Andrew nods. "Yeah, I've got it. I'll finish the chart here."

Rebekah's gaze shifts toward Micah's mother, asleep in the chair next to Micah. "She'll need to be briefed when she wakes."

"I know," he says softly. "I'll handle it."

He stares at the screen as Rebekah leaves, resisting the urge to scroll back through the data again. There is nothing new to find, but something in him still searches, still strains to find a pattern beneath the noise.

Next to his bed, Micah's mother, Lena Vasquez, dozes in a molded plastic chair, her body folded in the way only exhaustion allows. She wears dark jeans and a faded burgundy sweater, sleeves pushed past her elbows, as if she rolled them up hours ago and forgot. Her dark hair is pulled back in a low, loose ponytail, strands having long since escaped to frame her face. Concerns etch gentle lines around her mouth and eyes; creases developed from the weight she's carried for too long without rest. Standing alongside Micah's bed, Andrew takes in the scene. Lena rests one hand on Micah's bed as if reaching out to him while the other hand openly cradles her phone, which lights up with a silent alert from her school's attendance portal.

Andrew recognizes the app. His wife, Sonia, uses it almost every weekday morning to log late arrivals, absences, or reminders about early pickups. It's part of their rhythm, the quiet administrative choreography that comes with parenting a child who sometimes needs slower starts. Sonia works at Angelina Eberly Elementary, too. As a local school to the hospital, many doctors have family in attendance at or working for the school.

Sonia's an instructional lead who often floats between classrooms, co-teaching lessons, and mentoring new teachers while also supporting her own course load in mathematics. Her name carries weight in those halls, for the way she speaks to every student as if they are the only one in the room, and of course, for her solid curriculum skills. Andrew admires that about her, that blend of warmth and structure, the way she makes kids feel safe just by showing up.

Now here is Lena, someone Sonia speaks of with affection. She is a steady presence in the counseling office, the kind of colleague who keeps emergency granola bars in her drawer and thank-you cards in her purse. Sonia describes her as the quiet backbone of the school, the one who notices the kids who need additional recognition or emotional support.

Andrew remembers when Sonia first mentioned her. It was during a back-to-school night when they passed Lena in the hallway, bent over a student having a personal crisis. Lena calmed the child without saying much, using presence and patience. "She's the real kind of strong," Sonia said.

Andrew doesn't wake her. He envies her ability to rest, how she can fold into a plastic chair and find sleep amid the hum of machines and the sharp scent of antiseptic. More than the exhaustion; it's trust, or maybe the kind of resignation that comes when a parent has nothing left to give but hope.

Watching her now, Andrew sees a different side of the woman Sonia has spoken about so often. Today, Lena has stepped out of her role as the reliable counselor with an easy laugh. Today, she's a mother wrapped in quiet panic, doing what all parents do when the world tilts. She's surviving minute to minute.

Andrew turns his gaze back to the monitor. The soft rise and fall of waveforms move steadily across the screen, each pulse of light marking a moment of his patient's recovery. The measured, methodical work of a child's brain trying to find its footing again. Andrew adjusts the screen's contrast, slightly out of habit. For now, the data holds steady.

Micah twitches in his sleep, a slight movement of his hand that catches Andrew's attention. The seizure passed before he arrived, but something about the boy's EEG pattern continues to nag at him. Andrew wouldn't describe it as chaotic. Unusual in that rhythms and interruptions don't quite fit known syndromes. He makes a mental note to recheck the scans.

This isn't just another case. Micah's presentation carries echoes of other recent patients with similar bursts of unexplained electrical activity and no family history or prenatal red flags. The thought triggers a flicker of memory.

He is back in the ER six months ago. There was another child, nine years old, small for his age, eyes rolling back as the EEG danced with chaotic spikes. Andrew remembers the sharp smell of antiseptic, the hum of the same machines, and the frantic voice of that boy's father asking if it was something he'd done. The boy's labs were clean, his scans spotless, and still the brain misfired, waves twisting into patterns Andrew couldn't name.

In that moment, standing over Micah now, the sound of the monitor's steady rhythm folds into the memory's noise, the same irregular stutter of lines on the screen, and the same silence after the seizure passed. The familiarity sends a current through Andrew's chest.

He blinks the memory away, grounding himself in the present. Each time, Andrew ruled out the usual suspects, and each time the data whispered that he was missing something.

A noise in the hallway breaks Lena's sleep. She opens her eyes halfway, blinks at the machines, then looks at Andrew.

"How long was I asleep?" she starts, voice gravelly.

"Not long," Andrew says gently. "He's stable now. The EEG is trending toward normal. Micah's in good hands."

Lena rubs her face and sits up straighter. "You're... Andrew," she catches herself, adjusting her tone with a hint of embarrassment, "Dr. Turbin, right? My friend Sonia talks about you. I've seen your picture on her desk."

He smiles softly. "She talks about you, too. She says you're the heart of Angelina Eberly Elementary."

Lena laughs. "That sounds like her. I just try to show up. For the kids, you know?"

Andrew nods. "You showed up for yours. That matters."

She looks at Micah, then back at Andrew. "They keep saying they don't know what caused it. But something must have."

"I believe that too," Andrew says, more to himself than to her. He stands and makes one last check of the monitor. "Delta wave normalization," he mutters, jotting a note.

Sensing Lena's lingering worry, he motions her gently toward the monitor. "Here. Do you see these?" he asks, pointing to the waveforms. "These are Micah's delta waves. Earlier, they were chaotic and irregular. Now they're settling into a rhythm. That's a very good sign."

Lena's eyes are fixed on the screen. Andrew can see the lines between her brow crease and her eyes tighten. He's seen that look before and presumes that she may not fully understand what she's seeing.

"This line here is his brain starting to regulate itself again," Andrew explains. "The postictal state is the confusion after a seizure. It's easing. That's what we want."

Lena lets out a shaky breath. "So, he's really stabilizing?"

Andrew nods. "We're keeping him on Keppra, a medication that helps stabilize the brain's signals, reducing the risk of further seizures without heavy sedation. It acts quickly and is generally well-tolerated in children. We'll re-evaluate his neuroimaging in the morning, but yes. Things are moving in the right direction."

A hint of calm returns to her posture. Andrew observes Lena's brow relax and a gentle smile form at the edges of her mouth. It looks like belief is beginning to settle within her.

He checks the clock and curses under his breath. He turns back to Lena.

"The nurse in charge of Micah's recovery will check in with you shortly. She'll go over everything and give you the option of staying the night. There's a sleeper chair we can roll in if you need it."

Lena nods, visibly more at ease now.

"Also," Andrew adds, "Dr. Rebekah Cho is overseeing Micah's care tonight. She's the attending on call and has been with him since admission. I've gone over the consult notes and the scans with her, and she'll keep me updated if anything changes. I'll be back first thing in the morning to follow up." He offers a small, reassuring smile. "You're not alone in this."

Andrew makes his final entry in Micah's chart, recording that Micah's vitals look stable. EEG patterns have smoothed into a calmer flow. The Keppra infusion is holding. Andrew hesitates, pen hovering over the final note. He doesn't want to walk away. While the case doesn't require any more from him, not tonight, shifting his focus means stepping into another world. The world where he isn't the expert, just the dad who often shows up late.

He tucks Micah's chart under one arm while retrieving his cell phone from his pocket and taps out a message to Dr. Cho.

> Micah Vasquez. Seizure cluster. Improving. EEG trending normal. Stable on meds. Mother awake. You good to return?
>
> —A

Her reply comes quickly.

He allows himself a small smile. Rebekah never misses much. Andrew nods toward Lena and says, "I'll see you again in the morning." With that, Andrew heads for the elevator.

Stepping into the elevator, Andrew feels a familiar ache settle beneath his ribs. As he is removed from the clinical concern for a child in recovery, he moves instead into the raw ache of fatherhood pulsing just beneath his professional exterior. He often wonders how his colleagues with children handle it. How do they manage the separation between their white coat instincts and the parental dread that never really lets go?

Somewhere between Micah's age and his daughter's diagnosis, the line blurs for him. He tries to compartmentalize. He tells himself he can walk from a consult room into surgery and not carry a single image with him.

Andrew leans against the elevator wall, the soft whir of machinery humming through the silence. Theo Manning steps in, a tablet PC tucked under his arm.

"You all right?" he asks, glancing at Andrew.

Andrew hesitates before answering, eyes fixed on the floor numbers climbing overhead. "Every time I leave a room like that, I see Junie."

Theo's expression softens. "You mean you see her in them."

Andrew nods. "Every scan. Every uncertain case. It's like she's there, waiting behind the data. It's supposed to make me sharper, but some days…" He trails off, rubbing the back of his neck. "Some days it just feels like a bruise I keep pressing."

Theo studies him quietly, then says, "That's not weakness, Andrew. That's empathy. It's the part that keeps you from becoming a machine."

Andrew forces a faint smile. "Yeah. But sometimes it feels like it's pulling me apart." He once believed that medicine was a tool of certainty, a blade to cut through the fog of fear. Now he knows better. Medicine is a map, and too often, he traces it in the dark.

When the elevator doors open, Theo gives Andrew a nod of understanding before stepping out toward the opposite wing. "Get some rest," he says over his shoulder. Andrew raises a hand in acknowledgment as the doors close behind him.

A few floors later, the elevator dings softly, and Andrew steps out onto the first floor. He stretches briefly, feeling the shift from the enclosure of the elevator to the open corridor air. A nurse greets him with a nod as she wheels a cart past, and he murmurs a quiet goodnight. At the central desk, Andrew hands off Micah's chart to the charge nurse, summarizing the key points in a low voice. She listens, signs the handoff, and thanks him before turning to her next task.

Andrew lingers for a moment, watching the faint reflection of his face in the plexiglass divider. The hallway feels quieter now, just the distant pulse of monitors behind closed doors. He exhales, presses the elevator call button again, and after a brief pause, heads for the exit.

Outside, humid February air blankets the parking lot, thicker than he expected for this time of year. Living in Austin, Andrew knows too well that the weather never seems to follow the calendar. He slides behind the wheel of his car, replaying Micah's EEG, Lena's sleep-creased face, and the heavy silence of families who wait for a name to explain their child's unraveling.

Traffic near the hospital slows to a crawl. He considers calling Sonia to say he won't make it. Then he pictures his daughter scanning the crowd for his face, her paper crown tilting under stage lights. He runs the next red light.

He arrives at Angelina Eberly Elementary School well after sunset, the last hints of dusk long since swallowed by the dark. The parking lot glows with overhead lights, their halos catching swirls of dust kicked up by hurried footsteps. From the building's entrance, a low, audible buzz of laughter, applause, and the murmur of a packed auditorium between scenes. The building is a squat rectangle of aging brick and faded blue trim. It vibrates with the kind of evening energy unique to school performances. Parents hustle through the double doors, clutching phones and juice boxes, the smell of popcorn and poster paint trailing behind them. Inside, fluorescent lights cast a flat wash across the walls where hand-drawn signs and glitter-covered stars announce, "Welcome to the Kingdom of Kindness!"

The auditorium smells faintly of mop water and stage paint. Rows of metal folding chairs creak as people shift in their seats. A child sobs softly into a parent's sleeve. A volunteer usher, wearing a lanyard and a slightly wrinkled PTA t-shirt, intercepts him near the side door. "You can take the open seat over there. Quietly, please."

Andrew spots Sonia two rows ahead, auburn hair pinned with the same silver clip she's worn since grad school. She turns slightly, sensing him. Their eyes meet. No smile. No scowl. He takes it as a win.

Without hesitation, he slips past a few parents and quietly eases into the empty seat beside her. The chair groans in protest as he settles in, legs wobbling slightly on the uneven tile. Sonia gives him a sideways glance and a raised eyebrow but says nothing. Her expression says it all: *You made it.*

The curtain—a faded maroon divider—jerks open on its aging track.

The stage backdrop, a large colored castle drawn on butcher paper, sags slightly to the right. Spotlights flicker overhead, buzzing faintly. Their daughter stands a few steps left of center stage, aglow beneath the fluorescent wash, arms posed somewhere between a ballet flourish and a superhero landing. Her paper crown is prominent on her head. Her tunic clings backward, and her grin radiates defiance and joy.

"Greetings from the Kingdom of Kindness!" she declares, louder than the microphone can handle.

Laughter spreads through the gym. Andrew braces for it to turn sour, for an unwelcome giggle or an offhand remark that might overlook her joy and focus instead on her difference. He knows most of these families aren't unkind, just untrained. Sometimes, that's all it takes, a single look, a strained smile, or an awkward silence, to create a moment his daughter won't forget. He's seen it before. People around Junie hesitate, unsure how to respond when her sentences take strange turns, when she says something too big for her age, or when it is too abstract to follow. Those moments may not be meant with malice, but they can still hurt.

He sits on edge, his breath shallow, wanting to leap up and shield her from anything that might follow.

But nothing comes.

Just applause, real and sincere. For a moment, Andrew lets himself breathe. Junie, still center stage, beams beneath the lights like she belongs there. Because she does.

After the scene ends, Sonia turns her head. "She wrote that line herself," she whispers.

"Of course she did," he says, throat tight.

Later that night, Andrew and Sonia stand in the kitchen, each holding mugs of chamomile tea they don't plan to finish. Junie has been tucked in upstairs. She wore her crown all day at school and decided to wear it to bed as well, regardless of Andrew's concern that it might tear.

Andrew and Sonia now begin to close out their day. The tile floor is cold beneath their bare feet. The overhead light casts soft shadows across the countertop, cluttered with unopened mail, a sticky jar of peanut butter, and a piece of construction paper that reads "DAD IS A SCIENTIST" in marker and glitter.

"It sounds like she's still awake up there," Sonia says.

Listening for a moment, Andrew replies, "She's not. Just narrating her dreams again."

They smile. Sonia reaches for her phone, thumbs it open, then sets it down again without checking anything. "You want to play *Word Duel*?" she asks.

Andrew raises an eyebrow. "After the day I had? You'll crush me."

"Exactly." She grins and walks over to grab a pen from the junk drawer.

He chuckles and looks around the kitchen. His eyes settle on the science project their daughter left half-finished on the table, where paper planets are suspended with yarn and tape. "She's going to need a new hanger for Mercury."

"I told her not to use tape," Sonia says. "But she said scientists should test what fails."

"Actually, that's pretty accurate," Andrew replies with pride.

They smile again, the moment warmer now, lighter. Then the air shifts as Sonia leans on the counter, mug cradled in both hands.

Silence stretches between them, familiar and taut. Sonia breaks it. "You missed the first act."

"It was a seizure case. A little boy. I didn't think I could leave."

"You never think you can."

He doesn't answer. He reaches for scratch paper and a pen.

"What are you doing?" Sonia asks.

"His case was the same. No family history, clean prenatal scans. Still presenting with rare encephalopathy. And last week, there were two others."

"Andrew."

He stops writing.

"She's fine. She's healthy. Williams or no Williams. You don't need to decode her."

"I'm not decoding her," Andrew offers. "I'm trying to understand what's changing."

Sonia moves in close and places her hand over his. "I love that you're still looking. But don't lose the child you do have chasing the ones you couldn't save."

He nods. Expressing an acknowledgment rather than agreement.

They linger, still holding hands over ceramic mugs. The dog barks once upstairs, then quiets. Sonia tilts her head. "She asked me yesterday if her brain was broken."

Andrew blinks. "What?"

"I told her no. I said her brain makes a different kind of music. Just because it doesn't follow the same notes doesn't mean it's broken."

He exhales and presses her hand gently.

"We need to be careful," she adds. "With what we chase. With what we call abnormal."

Andrew nods again. He wants to promise her balance. Again, he finds himself wanting to be two people at once. Both the searching physician and the present father, the man who chases patterns and the one who can sit still beside his daughter's watercolor galaxies. No promise feels honest tonight. Only intention.

They move through the familiar rhythm of shutting down the house. Sonia flips the kitchen light off, drops a stray sock onto the laundry stairs, and locks the front door while Andrew unplugs Junie's glitter lamp in the hallway and turns down the thermostat. The dog has already claimed his spot at the foot of the bed, curled into a patient, lumpy sentinel.

Sonia brushes her teeth in quiet rhythm and changes into a soft, over-sized shirt that still smells faintly of lavender detergent. Andrew watches her move with tired grace, the day folding itself into her shoulders. When she climbs into bed, she reaches for her novel on the nightstand, a weathered paperback with a cracked spine and a ribbon bookmark holding her place. It's historical fiction, and she reads it slowly, one chapter at a time, claiming small pockets of peace where she can.

Andrew sits at the edge of the bed, rubbing the bridge of his nose. "I want to jot down a couple of notes before I forget," he says, glancing toward his study.

Sonia looks up but doesn't protest. "You always say that."

"And I always forget if I don't."

She smiles faintly and returns to her book. "Don't be long."

"I won't," he promises, though they both know he might be.

Andrew steps into his office. The room smells faintly of newsprint. He turns on the desk lamp, casting a golden circle of light over the scuffed surface. In the bottom drawer, his notebook waits. The Archive.

Andrew created his own dataset to record and track what he was observing with unexpected genetic anomalies in children. It began as a few loose pages tucked between case notes. He recorded the oddities that he couldn't let go of. Over time, however, it evolved into a sprawling, meticulously structured repository. He logged patient IDs, anonymized coordinates, birth environments, family histories, EEG charts, and phenotypic flags. Each entry included time-series observations, developmental milestones, and notations on early behavior shifts.

He used color-coded annotations to link common traits and developed a simple scoring index to rank unexplained severity. He tracked the emergence of variants of unknown significance (VUS) across disparate gene clusters and began noting when the same variant appeared across children with no shared background. His spreadsheet expanded into layered tabs, then into a private database he coded himself, allowing filters by date, geography, symptom onset, and genomic markers. For now, the Archive remained his alone. Andrew told himself it was caution; his data was preliminary, unverified, and easily misunderstood. He'd seen how quickly early findings could spiral through bureaucracy or the press before the science caught up. Better to wait until the signal was clear, until he knew what he was looking at, before inviting scrutiny that might bury the truth beneath procedure.

What began as pattern-hunting evolved into precise mapping. He gathered a dataset, and through that process, he created a lens. Through this lens, he began to notice a secondary signal made up of overlapping traits, early-onset hypotonia, atypical EEGs, and unclassified delays repeating in children with no clear genetic or environmental connection.

In that Archive, a quiet void emerged. Many children weren't showing signs of damage. They were showing signs of absence. Missing complexity. Subtle reduction in genetic expression without deletion. Variants labeled as "of unknown significance" became familiar, clustered, and then suspicious.

Opening the Archive now, Andrew flips to a blank page and writes:

Unnatural Patterns in Natural Variation?

Beneath it:

We keep looking for what's been added: pollutants, mutations, new stressors. But what if the real problem is not about what's added but with what's been removed? What if something essential is missing, and we're just beginning to see the consequences of that absence?

Then he draws a small square in the corner of the page. In it, he writes three words that capture the unease at the center of Micah's case:

Presentation Without Cause.

CHAPTER 3
SHADOWS IN THE DATA

The first rays of sunlight leak through the blinds in soft stripes, the smell of toasted bread drifts in from the kitchen, and the familiar sound of Sonia cheerfully humming fills the silence. From the kitchen, Junie narrates her procedure for putting cereal together as though hosting a cooking show, pausing only to ask whether queens eat granola.

Andrew stands in the hallway for a moment, with a coffee mug in hand, listening and cataloging each moment. Sonia and Junie are in the kitchen. He hears their laughter as Junie improvises a new recipe to try with breakfast this morning. The earnest hum of family life, steady and unremarkable in the best way. He remembers how quiet the house was before Junie spoke in stories, before Sonia showed him that routines weren't a trap, but a form of love.

He wanders in and rests against the doorframe. Sonia glances over her shoulder, wearing a sweatshirt he bought her years ago at a conference in Vancouver. Her hair is pulled into a messy knot, and waffle mix dusts one sleeve. Junie stands on a stepstool, one sock off, her crown of curls bouncing as she mixes something questionable in a bowl.

"Is that... pickles?" he asks.

Junie beams. "Almond butter and pickles. Like royalty!"

Sonia raises an eyebrow. "Your daughter."

"Our daughter," he corrects, smiling. "And clearly destined for culinary stardom."

He takes a sip from his mug. The coffee is a bit too bitter, but it doesn't matter. Junie's narrating again, something about a royal tea party and whether jellybeans can be used for diplomacy. Sonia listens with the same calm attention she gives to her students. She nods, offers questions, and gives Junie room to dream.

Andrew wants to stay in that moment, in the amber glow of safety and laughter. But the buzzing thread of unresolved questions tugs at his mind.

He glances at the clock. "I need to look at something before rounds."

Sonia nods. "You'll eat something first, though?"

He gives her a tired half-smile. "If there's any almond-pickle waffles left."

She laughs. "That one's all yours."

Andrew moves through the next several minutes on autopilot while his mind refocuses on work. He offers Sonia a quick kiss on the cheek. He takes a sip of her coffee by mistake, while Sonia gently corrects him that he missed one of the buttons on his shirt. These small rituals ground him.

Andrew plants himself at the dining room table and opens his laptop; the comforting haze of home life fades and is replaced by the cold glow of data and the unresolved tension curling in his stomach. He scrolls through Micah's EEG file again, dragging the cursor back and forth through the wave signatures. Then he opens another case, a girl from two weeks ago with a different presentation but eerily similar postical wave-forms. Then another, from last month. The patterns weren't identical, but they were etched in a code that he was attempting to decipher. Sharp peaks where there should be valleys. Recovery plateaus where there should be movement. The more he looks, the more echoes he finds.

He opens four EEGs side by side, highlighting anomalies. In the parietal lobe—the region that helps us make sense of touch, space, and movement—he spots short, uneven flashes of brain activity that don't line up in the tidy patterns doctors usually expect. Instead of the regular rhythms seen in known conditions, these bursts come in irregular spurts, as if the brain is skipping beats in its own internal song. This odd activity shows up after the seizure has passed, like a lingering echo, a neurological stutter suggesting the brain is holding onto the shock longer than it should, reluctant to return to its natural flow.

Andrew pulls his notebook closer and flips to the new patient log he began long ago. Children with neurological symptoms that resisted classification. Each case appears to carry the same haunting undertone. No clear cause. No family history. No warning.

He begins building a spreadsheet, populating columns for zip code, age, gender, presenting symptoms, birth hospital, delivery complications, vaccination timing, and even household income. The usual environmental suspects offer no consistent thread. No industrial clustering. No contaminated water overlap. The cases span neighborhoods, economic backgrounds, and urban versus rural distinctions.

He frowns and rubs his eyes. It's difficult to rule out an environmental or genetic factor without more research and subject profiles.

The door creaks, and Sonia steps inside, brushing crumbs from her hands. "I left the toast for Junie. She's trying another recipe for the almond butter and pickle spread. She thinks plain toast will work better."

Andrew makes a face without looking up.

She sets a mug down beside him. "Drink it before it goes cold. Again."

"Thanks," he murmurs.

She leans over his shoulder. "Still diving into brain squiggles?"

"Deeper than that. I keep finding these patients who don't match anything we know. Their genetics don't fit. Their symptoms vary, but there are similarities underneath. Something's shifting."

Sonia pulls out a chair and sits. "Do you think it's environmental?"

"I did. But the patterns don't hold up. It's not where they live, or what they eat, or even prenatal care." He taps a line on the screen. "Look at this EEG cluster. This is the more recent patient." Tapping another graph, "And this is the one from two weeks ago. Different hospitals. No known exposure to each other. And yet their brains show nearly the same recovery delay."

"So, what are you thinking?"

Andrew hesitates. He hates voicing half-baked theories. "I'm aware that all of my subjects so far have been children, and I want to make sure that's not skewing the data somehow. Still, it feels like something is missing. Something that failed to develop. Something they should have gotten, genetically, but didn't."

Sonia tilts her head. "Like a skipped step in a recipe?"

He smiles faintly. "Exactly. I want to go back and verify the absence of microplastics in the bloodstream. It's typically the first thing we check for idiopathic neurodiversity, but I want to review those notes again."

Sonia stretches back in her chair, watching him over the rim of her mug. "So, what's the next step? You chase this hunch until it's not a hunch anymore?"

Andrew runs a hand through his hair. "I don't know yet. Maybe I can gather more cases. Map them. See if the pattern holds."

"Do you think it will?"

He hesitates, staring at the closed laptop. "It's a feeling more than the data. Like I'm circling something just outside the light."

Sonia tilts her head. "Just promise me, when you go chasing it, you don't lose sight of what's already here."

Andrew reaches for her hand. "I see you. I see both of you."

She squeezes his fingers, then smiles. "Good. Because your daughter thinks jellybeans can end international conflict."

He laughs. "She might be onto something."

She taps his laptop. "Eat something. Then start looking at more recipes."

Andrew follows Sonia back to the kitchen, catching the clock again. The day is tugging at him, and he feels the anxiety that he hasn't made it to the hospital yet. It's the sense of obligation that competes with his desire to be present at home.

Sonia rinses out her mug, the clink of ceramic against the sink echoing lightly in the quiet. "Please remember," she says, drying her hands, "I start conferences this afternoon."

Andrew nods. "I'll make sure Junie gets picked up from school on time."

Andrew pours the last of his coffee into a travel mug. He kisses Junie on the crown of her curls, then turns to Sonia with a look that carries all the words he doesn't say: *I love you. I'm lucky you're mine. You're the best part of this life.* It passes between them in a glance, warm and certain. Then Andrew shoulders his bag and heads out the door.

Andrew takes a brisk, tolerable drive to Dell Children's Medical Center, the traffic flowing in a way that feels more like a concession than a reprieve. This is Austin, after all, where gridlock is less an inconvenience and more a civic identity. Still, for now, the congestion hasn't crested into its full crescendo. In thirty minutes, the same route will be gridlocked, brake lights stretching like a red river down every main roadway.

Andrew takes the temporary calm as a gift. He barely minds the traffic lights, his mind drifting to the EEG sequences he plans to recheck and Theo's promise to meet later. A song plays on the radio, but he barely notices it while his brain runs through his day and everything he hopes to accomplish with it.

Once he reaches the hospital, Andrew checks in with his staff at the neurology station. There's a short conversation with the night nurse and a quick scan through patient updates. Andrew gets a quick pat on the back from the attending doctor, who has covered early rounds, to let Andrew know that rounds have been covered. The familiar rhythm of the hospital kicks in almost automatically. The beeping monitors, the hushed voices, and the clipped footsteps on tile.

Before turning down the hall to the genetics wing, he makes a point to swing by Micah's room. Someone drew the curtain partway, and the glow of the EEG monitor lights the space in a gentle pulse. Micah lies still and peaceful, the twitch of his fingers gone. Lena sits in the same chair, now with a blanket over her lap and a paperback in her hand. Her eyes meet Andrew's as he steps quietly into the doorway.

"Good morning," he says softly.

She offers a small, tired smile. "Still stable. The nurse came by a little while ago to say the doctor on call would check in soon."

Andrew nods. "I'll be reviewing the imaging and EEG again this morning, just to be sure we're on track. You doing okay?"

Lena gives a small shrug. "Better. Seeing him like this... Better than yesterday."

He takes one last glance at the monitor. Delta waves are holding steady. Then he gives her a reassuring nod.

"Good," he says. "That's good."

Then he turns back into the hallway, the weight of her gratitude and fear trailing behind him like a shadow.

He moves quickly. He knows every corridor from the pediatric ICU to neurology, from genetics to diagnostics. The building hums with the steady current of activity. There are families in quiet clusters and nurses in crisp scrubs flowing like clockwork through glass-paneled hallways. Children's art adorns the walls, displaying crayon rockets, watercolor rainbows, and stick figures with stethoscopes.

Andrew doesn't often pause to notice the colors, but today he catches a glimpse of a finger-painted tree outside the elevator. Each leaf bears a name. He recognizes a few as former patients, some recovered, some not. He walks past it with a heavier step.

The neurology wing is quieter, tucked into a corner past the family resource room. Theo Manning works in the genetics lab down a narrower corridor. There's less color and more concrete. Andrew steps through the frosted glass door and finds Theo hunched over a monitor, a pen cap clamped between his teeth. Andrew pulls a rolling chair beside Theo's desk and drops a flash drive into the port.

"I need your help," Andrew says.

Theo stares back at him. "Always a good sign when you don't start with 'hello.'"

Andrew takes a breath. "I've been tracking a series of pediatric neurology cases," he begins, leaning in. "The last twenty-four months. All of them showed unusual EEG recovery signatures. Some demonstrated irregularities in the minutes to hours after the seizure ends. The brain recovery patterns look off, with lingering disruptions in rhythm and function that don't fit the usual post-seizure fatigue. I can't explain them. I went back and checked the genetic screens, and that's where it gets stranger. They don't align with known disorders, not even partial matches."

He pauses, gauging Theo's expression before continuing. "I want to focus on neurological presentations with unclear origins. Look at the screens that came back inconclusive or flagged VUS. I'm talking about the genetic junk drawer, the stuff we usually chalk up to statistical noise. But I don't think it's noise anymore. I think it's a signal we weren't trained to see."

Theo tilts his head, now fully attentive. "So, you think these VUS cases might share some underlying signature? Even if it's outside of the base sequences themselves?"

Andrew nods. "Exactly. Maybe it's in the expression. Or the suppression. A shift in what should be there but isn't. It's like the genome is improvising to fill a void."

"You going fishing? Chasing a thread that might unravel into something real, or it might just keep leading you deeper into the unknown?"

"No. This is targeted. There are too many cases showing drift from the expected phenotype. Something's gone slack."

Theo taps his fingers on the desk. "I can batch pull the sequencing files and run a similarity matrix. Maybe flag anything with sequence dropouts or unexpected methylation markers. But this is big. If you're right, we're talking about a new class of disorder."

Andrew nods. "Or a breakdown in how we transmit stability. Genetically speaking."

Theo jokes, "If this ends with you talking about cursed burial grounds or cosmic radiation, I'm out."

"Noted," Andrew says with a smile, but a part of his mind flickers with the word "burial." Maybe it's superstition, but he feels sure it's something else.

As Theo turns to his console, Andrew scribbles another note:

VUS recurrence: Check
Regions: Multiple. Non-overlapping

He underlines two words:

Unknown inheritance

Andrew's day unfolds in its usual whirlwind of rounds, check-ins, and another look at Micah's latest imaging. Time blurs, each task pulling him into the next. Before he knows it, the day has thinned to afternoon, and his watch buzzes sharply against his wrist. He glances down. *PICK UP JUNIE* flashes across the screen.

The walk to the garage feels short and long at the same time. His mind is working furiously while his feet handle the familiar motions.

By the time he pulls into the school's loop, Junie is already waiting with her backpack slung over one shoulder and a construction-paper magic wand in her left hand. She spots him before he reaches the curb and bolts for the car.

"Dad!" she yells, flinging the door open. "We had M&M math and I got seventeen!"

"Seventeen what?"

"M&Ms. But I gave two to Naomi because she cried when she only got brown ones."

He laughs, shifting into drive. "Smart and sweet. That's a good combo."

She grins. "And I drew Saturn with glitter."

"Of course you did."

As they pull away, Andrew glances at her in the rearview mirror, her sticky fingers, scuffed shoes, and constellation of freckles. She hums to herself, inventing a new melody as she counts the traffic lights.

The mystery of the day is still upon him. But for now, this moment is his anchor.

After they arrive home, Junie bounds inside, announcing her presence to the refrigerator and the dog with equal volume. Andrew helps her unpack her backpack, inspects the glitter-streaked Saturn, and pours her a cup of juice. At 3:45 sharp, the doorbell rings. It's Mandy, their sitter. Mandy's a college student with a gentle voice and a knack for art projects. Junie greets her like an old friend and immediately launches into the M&M saga.

Andrew lingers long enough to make sure everything is settled, then kisses Junie on the top of her head and slips out with a quiet promise, "Back by dinner."

The drive back to the hospital is quieter. His mind, briefly quieted by glue sticks and juice boxes, now snaps back to EEG clusters and inconclusive genomes. He is still chasing something. Still circling the same unanswered question.

By the time the sun dips behind the horizon, Andrew feels spent. The hum of Theo's server room still thrums in his ears, a heartbeat of unanswered questions. Data, patterns, and chemical traces blur together as he wrestles with Theo's challenge to read what the genome refuses to say aloud.

The drive home passes in a fog. He remembers the ignition, then the front door, but nothing in between. The familiar streets of Austin blur into ambient motion. His mind contemplates the data he shared with Theo. Data on signal drift and sequence gaps while they searched for overlooked clues. He pulls into the driveway and sits in silence for a moment, not quite sure how he got there.

Andrew steps inside and is greeted by the sound of laughter tumbling from the living room. Mandy looks up from a coloring book at the coffee table as Junie comes sprinting toward him, socks sliding across the hardwood floor.

"Dad! I showed Mandy my Saturn and we built a blanket tent and she let me use real scissors!" she announces, her voice climbing with each detail.

Mandy smiles from behind a stack of craft paper. "No casualties," she says with a wink. "She was a gem, as usual."

Andrew chuckles and drops his keys into the dish by the door. "Thanks, Mandy. I owe you a peaceful shift next time."

Junie tugs at his sleeve with impatient urgency. "Can we start dinner now? Chef Junie reporting for duty!" She dashes into the kitchen without waiting for an answer, dragging a chair across the floor as part of her ritual. After walking Mandy out, Andrew heads to the kitchen with a smile, already anticipating the chaos and the joy.

The kitchen fills with laughter, the percussion of vegetables being chopped, and Junie's running commentary on royal kitchen protocol.

Andrew lets her take the lead where it is safe to do so, offering gentle guidance between exaggerated stage directions and spice choices. They settle on fish tacos. Junie insists that cilantro is magical, but only when sprinkled with a "twirl."

As they eat at the table, Junie narrates the meal like a cooking show finale. He laughs, genuinely, as she offers him a taste of her "award-winning" pickle-lime salsa. For a while, it is just the two of them, the warmth of a shared meal, and the steady rhythm of a daughter who turns everything into a story.

Later, when the dishes are cleared, homework completed, and bedtime stories read, Andrew slips back into his study, green tea in hand. He scans his email and sees one from Theo. He opens the linked folder included in the email. A dozen anonymized case files wait for Andrew's review. Theo sent this batch to make sure he is pulling the right details.

Andrew begins reading. EEGs. Sequencing reports. Pediatrician notes. Observational charts. The first few files offer fragments rather than any breakthroughs. There are occasional overlaps, hints of shared delays, and uneven speech milestones. Developmental differences surface, but nothing yet forms a clear pattern. A few cases share auditory processing gaps, and others show speech onset regression. Each appears to have a clean family history. The files indicate that the doctors found no link to known disorders. It feels less like a revelation and more like the start of a long search, as if the genome itself pauses, uncertain how to fill in the missing lines.

Andrew reviews line after line and cross-compares clinical features. In several of the cases, faint echoes begin to surface. There are subtle irregularities that hint at shared disruption. Despite unrelated backgrounds, a handful of children in this small sample show mild variations in similar epigenetic markers, regions loosely tied to developmental timing and neurological pruning.

In relatively short order, he builds a three-column table:

- Child ID
- EEG Signature / Anomaly
- Missing Epigenetic Marker

He studies the chart for a long moment. Then, almost absently, he sketches a few rough circles in his notebook, trying to visualize where things might overlap. It's more of a hunch, a vague sense that something in these scattered details doesn't quite connect, like pieces of a map that may one day fit together but for now refuse to align.

He rubs his temples. Trying to stitch his thoughts together.

His mind continues to race. The pattern of absence gnaws at him, elusive and unfinished. Every name in his chart, every silent marker, points to a deeper thread that he feels compelled to tug free. The problem isn't what these children have; it's what they appear to lack. Something about that emptiness feels like an interruption and less like an error.

Andrew sits back in his chair, holding his notebook filled with underlined gaps and dead ends. The questions have evolved beyond clinical inquiries, becoming structural and generational. What if the problem isn't solely a genetic mutation or environmental exposure, but rather a malfunction in the inheritance architecture? What if specific traits aren't simply failing to be transmitted? What if they are being interrupted? It's a skipped sequence. A broken transmission. Perhaps the issue isn't limited to the genome alone. Maybe it involves the expression, or suppression, of something that was expected and is somehow absent.

He realizes, suddenly, that his search needs to reach beyond medical journals. If this is about transgenerational inheritance through the broader biological context, outside of DNA, then he should look beyond where clinical textbooks typically reach.

He opens a new browser tab and types: *transgenerational DNA inheritance*. The phrase has been echoing in his mind since he began wondering whether these children might be missing something that should have been passed down. If the genome is leaving out small pieces, maybe inheritance itself can falter. Most of the search results are vague videos, speculative articles, and conference slides. Then he finds a few unusual papers: one on changes to tissue DNA over time, another on microbial activity around burial sites. Finally, he notices a dense article from *The Indian Journal of Public Health Research and Development* titled, "Post-Mortem Genetic Cycling and Ecosystem Reintroduction in Humic Environments."

Andrew blinks. Ecosystem reintroduction?

He clicks. Scrolls. Scans.

One paragraph stops him:

Human remains interred in sterile, sealed environments fail to reintegrate genetic material into the local biome. Over successive generations, communities with high embalming and coffin-seal rates may inadvertently disrupt transgenerational genomic replenishment.

He stares at it.

Transgenerational genomic replenishment.

He picks up his pen and writes in capital letters:

GENETIC RECYCLING

The room feels colder. He stands, opens the biology text from med school, and flips to the decomposition section. It's a chapter he once skimmed for exams, never imagining he'd return to it in search of something so personal. The stages are familiar: autolysis, the body's own enzymes breaking it down from within. Putrefaction involves the invasion of bacteria and fungi, leading to the collapse of cellular walls. Finally, mineralization refers to the final redistribution of elemental matter.

Except it is the microbial pathways that hold his attention now. Fungi, bacteria, and archaea act as agents of decay, and more importantly, stewards of transformation. In the margins, he had once underlined a phrase: "the microbial bridge between organism and environment." These aren't just decomposers. They are integrators of organic material, carriers of fragmented DNA, and potential facilitators of horizontal genetic transfer. Could these ancient systems, so often dismissed as the final step, play a role in beginning again? Could they be part of what re-seeds the biome?

Andrew reaches for his notebook again, mind racing.

We expect inheritance to flow vertically, passed from parent to child through the coded strands of DNA. Yet not everything we carry is limited to that line of descent. What breaks down in the soil, like cells, microbes, and fragments of genetic material eventually reenters the living environment. Over time, it can influence the microbial communities that surround us and, indirectly, the life that grows from them. In this way, what came before doesn't vanish completely; it lingers in the ecosystem, folded back into the cycle that sustains us.

He turns to his Archive and writes:

If we block nature's return, do we cut off the cycle that sustains us?

CHAPTER 4
MEASURED IN MOMENTS

Sonia's day starts before the first bell. From the moment she steps onto school grounds, she follows the practiced rhythm of triage and care. As an instructional lead, she is expected to float between classrooms, co-teaching lessons, and mentoring new teachers while also supporting her own course load in mathematics.

Just after morning announcements, a fifth-grade student bursts into her office without knocking. His voice is sharp with panic. His backpack was stolen, or maybe it was just misplaced. Sonia crouches down, eye level with him, and slowly walks him through a few calming breaths. Within minutes, they retrace his steps, find the backpack two classrooms over, and return it to him. No scolding. No shame. Just the quiet restoration of order in a world that had briefly collapsed.

A few hours later, in the cafeteria, she notices a fourth-grade girl sitting alone, her tray untouched. Sonia joins her on the bench, starts with a question about the book she saw the girl reading last week, and waits. It takes time, but eventually the girl whispers that she feels invisible. Sonia nods gently and stays until lunch is nearly over. Before leaving, she hands her a Post-it note with a tiny doodle and the words: "You matter more than you know." The girl doesn't smile, not quite, but she folds the note like it's a secret she intends to keep.

She moves from classroom to classroom like a conductor managing a dozen moving scores. In Mrs. Patel's fifth-grade math class, she crouches beside a boy whose paper is covered in eraser smudges. "Walk me through your thinking," she says. He explains his steps, haltingly, and she nods, redirecting him with a quiet, "You're closer than you think. Try that middle step again." When he solves the problem, she taps the edge of his desk and grins. "See? You built that."

In the next room, a first-year teacher fumbles through a long division lesson that's quickly unraveling. Sonia steps in with easy calm. "Let's pause here," she says to the class, then models a new approach on the board, turning the problem into a story about sharing pizza slices. The students laugh and engage again, and the young teacher exhales in visible relief. "That's all you," Sonia whispers before leaving.

In Ms. Bennett's second-grade room, she joins a reading circle and kneels beside a boy clutching a worn copy of *Frog and Toad*. He hesitates, stutters on the first line. Sonia rests a hand lightly on the book. "It's just you and me right now," she says softly. "Let's give Frog a voice." The boy breathes out and tries again—slowly, steadily—and by the last page, his smile is as wide as the book itself.

Between classes, she spots a kindergartner frozen in the hallway, one shoe dangling from a broken strap. Sonia kneels, ties the loose end together with a teacher's practiced efficiency, and says, "There. You're faster now—go prove it." The girl takes off running, laughter chasing her down the hall.

Later, during her coaching block, Sonia finds a first-year teacher sitting slumped over a pile of ungraded papers. "They're sweet," the teacher admits, "but I feel like I'm failing them."

Sonia pulls up a chair. "You're not failing them," she says. "You're learning them. That takes time." Together they rewrite the lesson plan, cutting unnecessary steps, building in moments for breath and play. By the end, the teacher looks lighter, her shoulders less tense. "You'll get there," Sonia says with a reassuring smile. "You already are."

Sonia reassures her, then helps rework the lesson plan to better match the students' pace.

It's the kind of day that leaves her tired in a good way, mentally worn but proud of the work.

By the time the final bell rings, Sonia has taught two math blocks, led three coaching debriefs, helped calm students in tears, and answered no fewer than thirty emails from teachers, parents, and the assistant principal. She barely touches her lunch. Her reheated leftovers sit cold on the corner of her desk, next to a stack of ungraded exit tests. Still, the kids stay engaged, her teachers show progress, and no fire drills interrupt the momentum. By school standards, it's a win.

But the day isn't over.

As the thunder of 300 kids racing for the exit echoes through the hallway and the school day formally ends, Sonia feels the familiar tightening in her chest from the anticipation of what comes next. There's something about conference night that sharpens everything. A day of motion becomes an evening of meaning. Of exposure. Of facing the truths behind report cards and rubrics.

There are parents tonight who will ask her to help their child find the path back to something lost. There are others who won't realize anything is missing.

Even after years of doing this, Sonia still feels the weight of each conversation before it begins. Her role will shift from coach to confidante, from observer to interpreter. What she says in these next few hours may sit with some parents longer than anything they hear all year, and what they don't say may be even more important.

She presses her hands into the small of her back, stretches, and breathes in deeply.

Parent-teacher conferences begin at 4:30 sharp. She checks her notes, resets her brain, and shifts into the next role of listener, explainer, and advocate. Sonia takes a long sip of water and scans the schedule. The names blur for a second, and she blinks hard. It's going to be a long evening. She just hopes the tissues in the lounge aren't all gone yet.

As she makes her way to the teacher's lounge, the sharp fluorescent lights cast a pale, almost clinical glow over the mismatched chairs that have seen better decades. An old sign-up sheet from last fall's potluck still clings to the bulletin board. Sonia takes a moment to refresh her coffee and settle in at one of the tables. She sits alone and sips burnt coffee from a chipped mug that reads "WORLD'S OKAYEST TEACHER." It was a student's ironic gift she meant to toss but never did.

She glances over her schedule for the evening. Twelve families. Four back-to-back meetings. One student with two sets of parents. A few with none.

Her conferences will take place in room 114, a modular classroom just off the main building. She walks in, straightens the chairs, makes sure the whiteboard is clean, and lays out a small box of tissues on the table. A few of her colleagues think it's overly dramatic. Sonia knows better. She still remembers last year's spring meeting with Jordan Reyes' mother, when the woman sobbed after reading her son's writing journal. Sonia fumbled for napkins from her lunch bag because she hadn't brought tissues that day. Jordan's mother apologized between gasps, saying no one had ever shown her his writing before. Since then, Sonia has made sure to keep tissues on the table. It isn't about theatrics. It's about being ready when someone finally lets themselves feel something.

The first meeting was supposed to be with Lena Vasquez, but it has been postponed to a date in the future after Micah comes home from the hospital. Sonia did have a few moments with Lena earlier in the day when Lena swung by the school to pick up some of her personal items and her work laptop so she could keep up with emails and student assignments as time allowed. Lena texted Sonia to let her know that she was rushing in, and Sonia made it a point to be present when Lena arrived in her classroom.

Sonia recognized the fatigue behind Lena's smile the moment she walked in. She looked five years older than she did a month ago, and her eyes darted more than usual.

They hugged briefly, then held hands while Sonia hoped to shoulder some of the weight of what Lena must be going through. Sonia knew too well the feelings and emotional weight that Lena must be feeling.

"Thanks for making time," Lena said.

"Always," Sonia offered. "How's Micah?"

Lena exhaled slowly. "He's doing better, they say. The seizure appears to be isolated, but he hasn't quite come back. You know what I mean? He sleeps more. Says strange things. Sometimes he doesn't finish sentences."

Sonia nodded. "Andrew mentioned he saw him yesterday."

Lena smiled faintly. "Your husband is... Calm. It helps."

They talked for several minutes, the conversation easing into the small, personal details that parents and friends share when they both care about the same child. Lena's voice softened as she described Micah's endless curiosity and how he asks questions that leap from one topic to another as if he's following a secret thread only he can see. Sonia laughed quietly, adding her own stories about how Micah once spent an entire recess building a convoy of toy tractors in the sandbox, arranging them by size and color before assigning each a "mission." He gave the smallest tractor the most important job of delivering a pebble to a castle he'd made at the far edge of the playground because "Little tractors can do big jobs too." Lena's smile flickered at the memory, her eyes watered just enough to betray the emotion she was holding back, and for a moment, the two women lingered there in the comfort of recalling the Micah they both knew, as if speaking of him this way might keep him close while he finds his way back.

"He's still in there," Sonia said softly, offering a gentle smile. "Kids are resilient in ways that surprise us. Sometimes they step off the path for a while but find new ways forward. I've seen it. I believe Micah's finding his own way, just at his own pace."

Lena dabbed her eyes and nodded. She looked down at her hands for a long moment before speaking again. "I keep thinking maybe I missed something. Maybe I wasn't paying close enough attention."

Sonia touched her wrist gently. "Every parent thinks that. Especially when something unexpected happens. But I promise you, Micah knows you're here. That matters more than you realize."

Lena looked up, her eyes glassy. "He asked me this morning if his brain was broken."

Sonia's breath caught. She waited a moment and then asked, "What did you tell him?"

"I told him no. I said it's just figuring out a new rhythm."

Sonia smiled. "That's a beautiful answer."

Lena nodded again, more firmly. "We'll wait. However long it takes."

The meeting was quick, and Lena drew it to a close when she looked at her watch, saying, "I need to get back before the next check-in with the doctor. My sister is with Micah right now, but I know she needs to get back to work."

Sonia gave her a long embrace and offered to bring over a meatloaf once Lena and Micah are home.

With Lena giving up the first conference spot today, Sonia is hopeful that she can wrap up early. She pulls out her student progress folders and prepares to get started.

By the time the third family files in, Sonia feels her reserves slipping. Each conversation blurs into the next. Remarks on trouble focusing, anxiety spikes, and reading comprehension delays. It feels like more kids are struggling than usual. She knows it isn't just post-pandemic stress or overdiagnosis. Perhaps something deeper coils beneath the surface. Maybe Andrew's theories are rubbing off on her.

She thinks of a student from earlier in the semester. Naomi is a quiet girl who rarely speaks, but she once wrote a story so vivid it left Sonia breathless. The story is about a fox who forgets it's a fox and wanders through a forest trying to imitate the other animals. It watches birds sing, deer leap, and bears growl, but it feels out of place no matter what it tries. At the end, the fox curls into a den and whispers to the stars, wondering what it has lost. The story's final line read, "Some animals go quiet when they forget who they are." That line still affects Sonia.

Lately, Naomi has become more withdrawn, slower to raise her hand, and often forgets to turn in assignments. Nothing alarming, just enough to raise Sonia's concern. At the last conference, Naomi's mother seemed distracted from the start, clearly stressed and glancing at her phone between questions. She asked Sonia what she planned to do to get Naomi back on track.

"You're the teacher," she said with a polite smile. "She did so well last year. I don't know what changed."

Sonia gently suggested more reading time at home and fewer distractions. The truth, though, is hard to say. Naomi might be overwhelmed;

she might need something more than a checklist. Sonia can't diagnose or fix what she doesn't fully see. All she can do is keep the door open.

She nods, even as her stomach turns. Naomi needs presence more than a worksheet and homework. She needs someone to look her in the eye and ask what's going on at home. But Sonia can't do it all. Not for everyone. Not alone.

One father leans in halfway through the conference, after Sonia gently walks him through his son's declining reading scores, impulsive classroom behavior, and a sharp drop in vocabulary retention. She pulls up examples of work from the fall compared to more recent assignments, hoping to show a path forward. Yet, instead of asking about strategies or supports, the father goes quiet.

He rubs the back of his neck and glances at the door to make sure it's closed. Then he looks back at her, voice low and unsure. "Do you think there's something in the water?"

Sonia blinks. "What do you mean?"

"I mean—just—my son isn't the only one struggling," he says, eyes searching hers. "A couple of the kids on his soccer team seem off, too. They seem distracted. It's like they're having trouble keeping up, even with things they used to enjoy."

He shifts in his seat. "Sometimes I wonder if it's something subtle, like too much screen time, or maybe even the water. I don't know. I'm probably overthinking."

Sonia gives a slight, thoughtful nod, neither fully committing nor dismissing him.

He looks down at his hands, almost embarrassed. "I know it sounds crazy. You see them every day, though. Don't you notice it too?"

Sonia is unsure how to respond. She doesn't disagree with him. Part of her does agree. Instead, Sonia offers a small smile of acknowledgment, and the question lingers unanswered.

After all the parents have left, Sonia has a quiet ritual for closing out conference nights. She lingers in the classroom for a few minutes, resetting chairs, erasing the whiteboard, and letting the conversations settle before stepping back into the hallway. It helps her draw a line between the weight she carries inside those meetings and the life waiting for her at home. She learned early in her career that if she takes every child's struggle home with her, she won't last the year. So, she folds them gently into the edges of her mind and places them beside her lesson plans close enough to guide her while also far enough not to drown her.

Afterward, Sonia walks the hallway, saying good night to her colleagues. The posters on the walls advertise test prep boot camps and school pride rallies. A cartoon brain lifts weights. A banner reads: "Every Child Can Learn."

She stops and stares at it.

Standing there now, the words strike a discordant note against everything she's just heard. Last week, she sat with a student who couldn't articulate what was wrong, who said he felt like he was floating, like his mind sometimes left the room without him. A month before that, a mother broke down in the parking lot, telling Sonia she was too tired to argue about bedtime anymore, too overwhelmed to monitor screen time, too stretched to care the way she used to.

Sonia believes children can learn. But what happens when the world around them forgets how to support that learning? When families fray under pressure, and the systems meant to catch them grow thin?

She touches the edge of the banner as if to steady herself. The message feels incomplete, and in that gap between slogan and struggle, Sonia feels the ache of something honest, something unresolved.

The tools they use, including assessments, rubrics, and structured interventions, all feel mismatched to her students' needs. They are functional, but they seem broken or blunt. It's like trying to catch a storm in measuring cups. She senses gaps she can't name, feels most in the space between her instincts and her resources.

When she gets home, Junie is already asleep, the faint sound of her breathing drifting down the stairs like a lullaby left behind. The kitchen smells faintly of fish and garlic. Sonia steps into the soft light to find the table already set. Nothing fancy. Two plates of reheated fish tacos wait beside a small bowl of salad and a folded dish towel in place of napkins. A candle flickers between the dishes, half-melted and clearly borrowed from the bathroom counter.

Andrew had already eaten with Junie earlier. Sonia spots the telltale kid-sized plates in the sink and the crayon-labeled sticky note that reads, "Love you, Mama!" in Junie's looping scrawl. But he sits now with a second plate in front of him, untouched, waiting. He will eat again, just to keep her company. To make sure she doesn't sit alone at the end of a long day.

Next to Andrew is a stack of papers and his notebook open, one foot tapping lightly under the table like he's still working out a puzzle in his head.

"Surprise," he says, a little sheepish. "It's just leftovers, but I thought..."

Sonia smiles, the kind that makes the weariness pull back just a little. "You thought right."

Sonia drops her bag and pours a glass of wine.

Andrew stands up as she walks closer and pulls her into a big, loving embrace, wrapping his arms around her like he can shield her from everything she's carried home. She lets herself sink into it for a moment, breathing in the comfort of garlic, candles, and familiarity.

"How are you feeling? How were the conferences?" he asks, still holding on gently, his voice low and full of care.

They sit together, and she lets her shoulders sag. "It's subtle, but I'm noticing more students struggling to keep pace. They struggle academically and emotionally. Gaps in focus, slower problem-solving, and less confidence. It's not all at once, and not everyone, but it feels like... Something's off."

"I get it," Andrew agrees.

A small smile pulls at the corner of Sonia's mouth. "Maybe I've been spending too much time listening to your theories," she says. "Maybe I'm just adopting your concerns and projecting them onto my own students. Seeing things because I expect to."

"I think about that too," Andrew offers. "All the time. I mean, my job is crisis. I see kids when something's already gone wrong. That's the only lens I get most days." He pauses, his voice softening. "It's easy to forget how many kids are okay. Resilient. Thriving, even. It's just hard to see that when all I handle are the exceptions. We have to remind ourselves that the few can't define the whole."

"Still, the few are asking for something," Sonia says, glancing at his notebook before continuing, "How about you? Did you get anywhere with your notes today?"

Andrew gives a half-shrug. "Some. It's like trying to hear a melody in a room full of echoes," he says. "There's something recurring in the data, slightly delayed problem-solving sequences, slower word recall… but it's faint. Faint and inconsistent. Like a shadow that disappears when you try to chase it."

He pulls his notebook a little closer. "I started thinking about it like harmonic distortion, when multiple signals overlap and interfere with one another. You can't always separate which sound is intentional and which is interference, but if you track the waveform long enough, a pattern starts to hum underneath it. That's what I think I'm seeing. It's subtle, barely noticeable. Hardly a whisper. Just a presence. Something quiet but real."

Sonia raises an eyebrow. "You and your metaphors."

"Hey," he says, smiling, "they work. At least for me. I started sorting out what might be signal and what's just noise. There's a pattern… maybe. But it's early."

She reaches for his hand. "You'll see it more clearly tomorrow."

He gives a small smile, grateful. "Yeah. Maybe I just needed a dinner break with you."

They don't say much more after that. They sit at the table, slowly making their way through dinner, sharing the bottle of wine Andrew opened earlier. The silence between them is companionable, a kind of quiet reserved for people who have carried enough words all day and simply want to exist in the presence of someone who understands. Sonia lets her head rest in one hand for a moment, eyes closed, while Andrew absentmindedly traces the rim of his glass with his fingertip. They don't need to speak to feel heard.

CHAPTER 5
MISSING BLUEPRINTS

Dr. Meera Rao stands out in any room because her presence invites attention without demanding it. She draws people in through quiet conviction and composed attentiveness. There's a quiet clarity to her presence, the kind that makes people lower their voices and listen more closely. Her dark hair, threaded with the first signs of silver, is pinned into a practical bun that never quite stays put. A single curl always escapes to rest against her cheek. She wears minimal jewelry, including a delicate chain at her neck and a copper bracelet on her right wrist. Most days, she adds a scarf, usually cotton, draped loosely over one shoulder in homage to her grandmother's habit of doing the same.

She's tall for a woman in her family. Her eyes are deep brown and serious, framed by the kind of creases that come from years of reading case files under dim clinic lights, testaments to a life of rigorous observation. At first glance, people may mistake her for an academic. Upon a second glance, they realize she's something more; she's an observer of biological, cultural, and environmental systems.

Meera Rao is a pediatric clinical researcher affiliated with a government hospital in Hyderabad, a city that sits at the intersection of India's layered histories and accelerating future. Hyderabad, Telangana's capital and largest city, is now a hub for India's booming tech and biotech industries. The city is a living collage of Mughal-era palaces, high-rise buildings, bustling bazaars, and gleaming research centers.

The pulse of Hyderabad beats with contradictions: ancient and modern, crowded and quiet, slow and sprinting. For Meera, it's the perfect base. It's rich with intellectual resources and still close enough to the rural communities where her questions live. Her office window overlooks a tangle of terracotta rooftops and satellite dishes, temples and tea stalls, all pressed together in the city's chaotic elegance.

Her current research focuses on congenital defects and regional genetic anomalies, particularly those that emerge in remote districts often overlooked by large-scale studies. In one such case, Meera traveled to a village in the Gadchiroli district after local midwives flagged an increase in cleft-palate births over the past decade. What struck her wasn't just the data, but the stories behind it.

She remembered visiting a home on the edge of a rice field, where a mother cradled a quiet, wide-eyed infant with a small ridge splitting the upper lip. The father, a weaver, had constructed a makeshift crib from repurposed bamboo and chicken wire, lining it with turmeric-stained cloth that smelled faintly of camphor. The family had no running water and no history of congenital illness. Meera sat cross-legged on the courtyard floor, sipping sweet lime water from a clay cup as she asked about prenatal care, family history, soil quality, and farming inputs. She watched as the grandfather knelt beside a well and explained, in hushed tones, how rituals had changed after the sacred grove nearby was partially cleared for road access.

The midwife mentioned that she'd delivered several similar cases in the last two years, all within walking distance of that grove. Meera collected soil samples near the homes and within the grove's perimeter. She noted the shift in vegetation, the thinning of the neem trees, and the absence of tulsi plants, which were once abundant in the area. Her report on the village was never published. Too little statistical power, too many unmeasurable variables. Still, she kept the file. It sat on her shelf with a yellow tab labeled, "Bhaskarwadi – intuition unresolved."

She's become a quiet expert in patterns others overlook, especially the ones dismissed as statistical noise. Where other doctors see rare conditions, she sees questions no one has asked yet. Her work crosses the boundaries between genetics, culture, and the environment, drawing on medical knowledge, deep listening, and respect for the histories carried in each village she visits.

At her desk, Meera sits beneath the rattle of an old ceiling fan. The fan has a slight wobble, like it might spin off its hinge in protest. Her desk is a collage of work in progress, charts spread out in loose arcs, plastic vials labeled in her careful script, and several dog-eared notebooks with scribbled marginalia.

Some of the surveys stacked beside her she'd led personally, navigating narrow village paths in worn sneakers, clipboard in hand, shaded by a scarf that doubled as both her sun cover and notepad protector. She prefers the field to the lab. Even now, surrounded by data, she can hear the voices of the women she's interviewed, the clang of borewell pumps, and the laughter of children in dusty courtyards.

It's messy, it's hot, and she loves it. It's where she feels most useful, like she's making a real difference.

For Meera, this isn't just work. It's personal. She grew up in the village of Shendurwadi, two hours east of Pune. It was a place where health, soil, and memory were all one ecosystem.

Meera was especially close to her grandparents. Her grandfather, a gentle man with a scholar's patience and a mason's hands, died when she was seven. Even in those short years, he taught her to listen more than speak and to observe the natural world with curiosity and care. Her grandmother, sharp-witted and steady, carried the family through his loss with dignity. She passed down the old herbal traditions, showed Meera how to tell the health of the soil by the way it crumbled in her palm, and made evening tea a daily ritual of presence and connection.

Her parents, both educators, nurtured her intellect with quiet intensity. Her father, Ravi Rao, taught mathematics at the local secondary school and viewed numbers as meaningful frameworks for understanding fairness and justice, beyond simple abstraction. He had a calming presence in the classroom, known for his steady voice and sharp chalkboard diagrams, and often brought his puzzles home, scribbling equations on the backs of receipts and cereal boxes for Meera to solve. He believed discipline lived in the details and that every problem could be unraveled with patience, no matter how complex.

Her mother, Malathi, taught language and civics at the same school and approached her work with equal passion. She instilled in Meera a reverence for stories, from literature to the narrative threads woven through laws, rights, and identity.

Their modest home was filled with paperbacks and the scent of roasted cumin. Dinner was rarely eaten in silence. Instead, it was a time for spirited debate, questions that challenged assumptions, and storytelling that stitched their days together. Questions were never discouraged; in fact, they were welcomed with enthusiasm. Her parents believed knowledge had power when paired with purpose and humility.

Today, her eyes are fixed on a dataset that's been bothering her for weeks. She first noticed something off during a peer meeting two months ago. A visiting epidemiologist presented regional birth defect maps as part of a standard comparative study. The room was only half-listening. Most of them had seen similar heat maps a hundred times before, but something in the color gradient caught Meera's attention. A faint blotch of red, just a shade darker than the rest, hovered over Bhira. Meera couldn't move past it, even when the presenter did.

She approached him afterward. "Was that Bhira?" she asked, pointing to a corner of the printout.

"Yes, I think so. Why?" he replied.

"That region's usually neutral," she said, narrowing her eyes.

He shrugged. "Probably a reporting anomaly. Small sample size."

Meera's gut told her otherwise. That single shade shift led her back through layers of her own field data. Patterns began to pulse faintly, like a warning light too dim to be noticed at first glance.

She looks at the line graph in front of her for what feels like a long time, trying to decide if the change she's seeing is real or the sort of drift she's learned to ignore.

The rise is less than half a percent, but it repeats across every district she's tracked, and that symmetry unsettles her. In three years of running this data, the curve has never bent in the same direction twice without cause. Random error doesn't align that neatly.

Most analysts would smooth it away, hidden in the rounding of larger models. But her method—hand-built and stubbornly precise—lets the noise breathe. It's in that thin breath of variance that she finds the beginning of something that shouldn't exist.

Meera reviews the incident reports and summary tables, dissecting the data layer by layer. She applies regression models to isolate variables, filters the samples through epidemiological software she's customized herself, and even cross-references physical soil samples she's collected from around birth homes. Her analysis encompasses dozens of potential confounding factors, including water contaminants, crop rotation, pesticide drift, and air quality. She pulls satellite vegetation data to look for signs of ecological disruption and pairs that with birth weight logs, clinic records, and community health worker notes written in hurried Marathi.

The conditions appear across different families with no clear genetic link and across communities that share neither a common water source nor similar agricultural practices. She runs allele frequency distributions across affected families and finds nothing connecting them beyond basic regional ancestry, which is far too broad to explain what she sees. She looks for clusters around industrial zones but finds none. She compares maternal age, education, diet, and prenatal care. Still, no consistent factors emerge.

The anomalies range widely, including cleft palates, limb malformations, and neural tube defects. Some are visible at birth; others emerge in the first six months. In isolation, each case appears to be an unfortunate event. Taken together, however, they form a low hum beneath the data, a pattern of disruption so subtle it would go unnoticed to anyone looking for a loud signal. Meera isn't. She learned to hear what others filter out.

Not all disruptions announced themselves in bone or skin. Some, she suspected, might live deeper in the neural scripts written before birth, waiting years before revealing their silence.

What truly catches her attention is the timing. The rise in congenital anomalies follows a slow, steady incline. It began in the 1980s, accelerated through the 1990s, and became unmistakable by the early 2000s. Over the last decade, the trend has intensified into a consistent, visible rise. The increase doesn't align with changes in diagnostic technology or health worker reporting methods. The arc of the data follows its own quiet rhythm of cumulative disruption.

Meera layers older paper records with newer digital reports and runs adjusted historical trendlines to verify the trajectory. The slope holds steady. It follows no seasonal rhythm and reveals no random variation. Conversely, it deepens over time.

The affected communities all share more than just proximity to traditional burial grounds. They border rivers, farmland, and forests shaped by centuries of ritual, migration, and survival. Some used sealed tombs; others returned their dead directly to the soil. A few, curiously, practiced hybrid customs of ceremonial cremation with partial burial of ashes in earth plots. Yet, burial practices aren't the only common thread. Meera traces dietary shifts, soil acidity, groundwater variance, and even changes in local flora. It's everything combined, or perhaps it's how all these elements converge. The deeper she looks, the less certain she becomes of the origin point. It's a puzzle with too many hidden corners, and the pieces refuse to form a clear picture. She can't shake the feeling that something fundamental has shifted.

One village health worker mentions that families living closest to the ceremonial forest near Bhira have higher reported rates of birth complications. Initially, Meera suspects reporting bias or data entry inconsistencies, but field interviews and clinic logs confirm the trend. These families are experiencing isolated complications including low birth weight, incomplete neural development, and rare craniofacial malformations. The health worker admits these conditions have slowly increased over generations, but no one has formally tracked them until Meera began asking questions.

What puzzles her most in this particular case is the absence of obvious causes. There have been no new factories, no change in water quality, and no major agricultural shifts. The infrastructure has, if anything, improved, but outcomes have worsened.

Meera jots a note in the margin:

No common exposure. No common ancestry. There is common proximity.

Then she sets her pen down and stares at the page.

The implications tug at the edge of her composure. If proximity is the connecting thread, then the source might be something rooted deeper than any known exposure. It might be something historical or sacred. She thinks of the burial grounds again, unmarked and unwatched. What if those sites, long believed to be peaceful endpoints, are instead quiet origins of disruption?

Her stomach tightens. She's following more than the data. She's stepping into a conversation no one wants to have. If she's right, it could unsettle entire communities, challenge cultural norms, and call into question decades of scientific silence. And if she's wrong…

She rewrites the note beneath the original, crossing out her earlier speculation. The new entry is concise, impersonal:

~~No common exposure. No common ancestry. There is common proximity.~~

Follow-up: compare anomaly frequency by gestational timing; evaluate correlation with methylation drift.

She sits back. It says what she means, though what she means feels larger than the words allow. She looks again at the gently rising line on the graph. Something is happening, and it's happening quietly.

The defects aren't clustering in typical ways. Meera ruled out environmental pollutants and known hereditary factors. Still, something's off.

She glances at a photo of her mother tacked above her desk. "Amma would say I'm chasing ghosts," she murmurs.

Meera's learned to trust the data, and this data whispers a pattern.

She clicks open a new file and begins typing a note to herself: "Compare community defect rates by proximity to preserved burial grounds. Control for embalming, interment method, and soil porosity."

Below that, she adds: "What are we introducing or keeping from the earth?"

The fan overhead clatters once, then steadies. Meera keeps typing.

This is only the beginning.

CHAPTER 6
GHOSTS OF THE SOIL

The road to Chikhalgaon unspools ahead of Meera and her driver, winding through rust-colored hills and fields of late-season millet that shimmer in the sunlight like golden fringe. The monsoon passed weeks earlier, leaving the landscape alive, the earth still breathing in slow exhales of moisture. Meera sits in the back seat of the government-issued Jeep, her satchel pressed against her side, a notebook balanced on her lap, and one hand gripping the overhead rail with practiced steadiness. The driver, Ganesh, keeps a steady hand on the wheel and an eye on the road, occasionally swerving to avoid potholes or goats that meander too close to the shoulder. He doesn't ask questions. Meera appreciates that. She's made this kind of journey countless times before. The rhythm of the road becomes its own kind of meditation, with the way the horizon dances beyond the windshield.

She isn't visiting the village for routine data collection. As the Jeep winds closer to Chikhalgaon, Meera feels the familiar churn of anticipation and dread. A part of her hopes to find nothing, that this visit will end in reassurances and explanations grounded in ordinary science. Another part, quieter and deeper, suspects she's already passed the coincidence threshold.

Her gut tells her she's pursuing more than a lead; she's chasing something foundational. If what she suspects is true, if burial practices and proximity to interred remains are influencing mutation rates, then her work may be crossing a line between observation and provocation. She wonders whether she's prepared for the consequences of being right, or for the ridicule that might come if she's wrong.

A whisper of self-doubt surfaces. Maybe the fatigue of too many sleepless nights parsing datasets yields more questions than answers. Perhaps it's the memory of her mentor, Dr. Halvorsen, who once warned her not to let patterns become poetry, not to mistake the symmetry of chance for evidence. Meera has never been afraid of the liminal spaces between disciplines. She worries that she's no longer standing at the edge of something unknown but already in it.

Two days earlier, Ramesh, one of the field nurses stationed at the Buldhana regional clinic, called with a tone she immediately recognized. The sharp-edged uncertainty arose when familiar symptoms began to behave in unexpected ways. Ramesh had sent the field summaries— numbers she had hoped would flatten but instead climbed again. She called it a late bloom, though that made little sense. The conditions hadn't changed, yet the anomalies were rising as if something buried years ago had finally reached the surface.

Ramesh commented that perhaps all any system needs is time. Maybe it takes years for small absences to add up and for the loss of one input to ripple outward until the balance gives way. The data don't prove it yet, but the curve feels less like a long-delayed echo.

A sharp pothole brings her back to the moment. The Jeep bounces past grazing cattle, a woman in bright saris carrying bundles of wood, and hand-painted signs that mark the village borders. Chikhalgaon appears like a watercolor emerging from a blank canvas. The air carries a warm, earthy scent laced with distant smoke and the tang of sun-warmed iron. The dusty road grows narrower with each turn, hemmed in by marigolds and bougainvillea spilling over worn stone walls.

Overhead, crows caw lazily from thatched rooftops, their calls mingling with the sharp crack of a cricket ball against a wooden bat in the distance. The rhythm of life is unhurried while purposeful.

Children run barefoot through the lanes, their laughter ricocheting off clay walls. Their voices rise and fall with the breeze, and Meera finds herself listening more than observing, letting the cadence of the village sink into her skin. She steps down from the Jeep and closes her eyes for a breath, letting the chorus of sights and sounds settle like layers of a story, ready to be read.

The clinic lies just past the village center. It's a square concrete structure painted in what was once a vibrant blue, now dulled and chipped by time and monsoon. A rusting water tank teeters beside it, perched on stilts and casting a long shadow over the cracked flagstones of the porch.

The rise in congenital anomalies has followed a slow, steady incline since the 1980s. Fast forward to today, and the trend has sharpened into a consistent, visible climb.

A nurse recognizes Meera from a prior visit and greets her with a soft "Namaste." Her name is Sunita, a compact woman in her late forties with a precise, no-nonsense manner. She wears her white uniform crisply pressed, with a pale pink dupatta folded neatly over one shoulder. Meera remembers her well. On her last visit, Sunita stayed late to help her copy birth records by hand when the electricity failed. They worked by lantern light at a back table, sharing stories over hastily brewed tea and the sound of distant crickets.

Today, Sunita brings tea again without being asked, sweet and milky, served in a steel tumbler still hot to the touch. She places it on the desk with a nod, already turning to fetch the files Meera requested.

Meera sets the tumbler beside a metal desk already laid out with a stack of birth logs, prenatal charts, and handwritten community health records. Some are bound in twine, others folded and marked in ballpoint ink, the paper worn thin in places from handling. She scans through them slowly.

She came to Chikhalgaon to review the files and to get a sense of the place. She wanted to be present and to observe the patterns that only emerge when you watch how people move through their day. She listens for those quiet gestures: a mother kneeling to retie her daughter's fraying sandal, a boy offering his last piece of jaggery to a coughing neighbor, an elder pausing at the threshold of a banyan grove to whisper a greeting into the air before stepping forward. They shape how Meera *sees* the data. They ground her observations in human experience.

Without that grounding, she knows her research risks becoming sterile, technically sound but spiritually adrift. The numbers here echo what she's seen in Bhira. There's a steady uptick in congenital anomalies just subtle enough to be dismissed by the casual observer but unmistakable to those who know where to look.

After two hours of meticulous review, she steps outside to stretch her legs. The sun has climbed higher, casting harsher light against the clinic wall. Under the porch's narrow band of shade, an older man waits, sitting cross-legged on a woven bench that sags gently under his weight. He's wearing a white kurta that has softened from years of washing, and a weathered Nehru cap perched slightly off-center on his head. His face bears the kind of lines that speak of seasons, sun-etched, wind-creased, and marked with the patient erosion of a life spent outdoors.

Sunita follows Meera outside, and noticing her gaze, Sunita introduces Meera to the man sitting on the bench. Dada Jalam, one of the village elders. He heard Meera was asking about births and about the forest.

"It used to be," he says in Marathi, voice slow but strong, "that when someone died, the body returned to the land. The Earth knew how to take care of its own. There was rhythm to it. Respect. We did not need much to say goodbye."

Meera nodded, listening intently. "And now?"

He looks away, his eyes scanning the hills beyond the village. "Now, we build boxes. Coffins. Concrete chambers. We close the bodies up. Seal them like secrets. And the Earth... the Earth is left out."

He pauses, then adds with a touch of sadness, "Some families don't even leave the dead in the earth anymore. They keep them in jars on shelves in their homes or in family chambers at the big cemetery near the highway. They say it keeps the memory close. But I wonder, if the earth forgets what it cannot reclaim, then what happens to the memory we hold apart from it? What happens to the circle we broke?"

She pauses, letting the words settle before scribbling the phrase in her notebook. "Seal them like secrets," she repeats under her breath, as if trying to understand what was being kept hidden.

Dada taps a weathered finger on the wooden frame of the bench. The motion is slow and deliberate, as if anchoring his words in the grain of the wood. Meera watches his hands—lined, callused, and confident—and feels something shift within her. It's more than curiosity. It's reverence. A sense that she is being entrusted with a knowledge older than her field-work, older than her tools.

She wonders how many stories have been lost simply because no one thought to ask, or worse, because they asked too late. Dada's words crack open something in her. The humility to accept that there might be truths science hasn't yet designed instruments to measure.

This is more than oral history. It's lived cosmology. For the first time in weeks, Meera feels less alone in her questioning. She realizes that what she's chasing in charts and soil samples might already live in the memo-ries of people like Dada, guardians of rhythms that the modern world has forgotten to hear. "My grandfather used to say that the land carries what it's trusted with and forgets only what's withheld. If we keep too much from it, then something is lost. It's lost piece by piece over time. The old ones believed that when a body returned to the earth, its essence spread through the roots and soil. That it traveled through the grain, the rain, the grass the cattle fed on. That life recycled in substance, more than in spirit. We would become the trees, the crops, and the animals who grazed the fields. We were part of the next breath and the next harvest."

He looks toward the hills again, eyes narrowed. "But now? We seal bodies in boxes or keep the ashes on shelves. We carry the memory, but not the body. We want remembrance without return. I think the earth notices. I think it hungers for what we no longer give back."

"Have you heard of sky burials?" Meera asks. Her tone is light, but she leans forward just slightly.

He smiles faintly, a flash of amusement in his eyes. "Yes, but not here. That is for mountains. For places where the birds fly closer to heaven. We had something like it, long ago. We burned the bodies on tall pyres, open to the sky. Not behind walls, not under cement. We believed the wind helped carry the spirit. That the ash fed the earth. That the memory of the person returned through the roots."

Meera closes her notebook gently and looks up. "When did that change?"

"After the school came. After the roads. After people with good intentions brought cement and donated coffins. They wanted to help. They didn't mean harm, but we stopped trusting what we knew. We stopped asking why we did things the old way."

The breeze stirs through the trees, lifting a corner of Meera's scarf. She stands and thanks him, her voice soft with sincerity. Then she pauses, her hand still resting on her notebook.

"When I was a girl," she says, "my grandmother used to compost everything. Food scraps, dried flowers from the prayer room, even the ashes from our cooking fire. She said the earth didn't just need water; it needed stories. And everything we returned to it, even in the smallest way, carried a piece of who we were."

Dada Jalam's expression is inviting, his eyes reflecting a quiet recognition.

"After she died," Meera continues, "we scattered her ashes beneath the neem tree she planted when she was sixteen. Every spring, it still blooms the brightest in the village. My father swears the soil remembers."

She smiles and nods again. "Your stories aren't forgotten. They're carried, too. I promise you that I will share what I learn."

He nods once as a gesture of trust, and perhaps more, he grants permission.

Back inside the clinic, the afternoon light stretches long across the tiled floor. Meera returns to her seat and finishes reviewing the last of the files Ramesh left for her. One chart stands out. It describes a child born with neural tube defects, with no family history and no apparent malnutrition. In another, she finds a chromosomal microdeletion—a sliver of missing code—invisible under a microscope yet capable of rewriting an entire development path. She adds both to her growing list, underlining one phrase again and again: no known cause.

She thanks Sunita, who's tidying up a corner cabinet, and shares a few final thoughts about follow-up care, data access, and the children's nutritional profiles. They agree to coordinate with the district office for additional screenings, though both understand how long that can take. As she steps toward the clinic door, Sunita presses an extra stack of community health records into her hands. "In case something small becomes important later," she says.

Meera nods, grateful. She tucks them beside her notebook and glances once more at the quiet rhythm of the waiting room, the worn benches, the posters curling slightly at the edges, the child tracing circles with her finger on the dusty windowsill. It's a small place, but it carries the weight of many lives.

She walks back toward the Jeep, the clinic behind her, and the burial forest in the distance. Meera looks out across the horizon. The forest stands in stillness, its canopy unbroken. Once, rituals here united generations; now they feel unobserved, separated from what they once served. The stillness settles in her chest. She wonders what trace remains when the exchange between the living and the soil is cut off, whether the system adapts or simply goes dormant.

She takes a long breath and turns back toward the road, wondering out loud, "If memory lives in the soil, what happens when we bury it in stone?"

The drive back to Hyderabad unwinds in silence. The sun dips behind the hills as the jeep hums steadily along the narrow road, its tires stirring fine trails of dust that catch the amber light. Meera rests her head against the window. Her scarf is tucked beneath her cheek. Notebook resting closed in her lap for the first time all day. The steady rhythm of the road feels heavier now. It was more than fatigue. It felt like the weight of too many threads beginning to tie together. She replays Dada Jalam's words, the grainy edges of the clinic files, the stillness of the burial forest. Patterns nudge at the edge of understanding, refusing yet to form a single picture.

Ganesh doesn't interrupt her thoughts, only glancing in the rearview mirror from time to time as the sky darkens and the city lights begin to glow on the horizon. By the time they pass the outer ring road and pull through the hospital compound gate, the evening has settled into its final hush. Meera gathers her notes, thanks Ganesh with a tired nod, and steps out into the thick, humid city air. Her legs ache from sitting too long, but her mind is already moving faster than her steps.

She climbs the hospital steps slowly, the weight of her bag pressing into her shoulder, the dust of the day still clinging to her sleeves. Inside, the air conditioning greets her with an abrupt chill, a stark contrast to the thick dusk outside. Her sandals echo softly down the polished corridor as she makes her way past familiar markers. Past the mural painted by pediatric patients and the cluster of shoes outside the meditation room. Nurses nod as they pass, their pace brisk and purposeful.

She doesn't stop at her department's front desk. Instead, she just lifts a hand in acknowledgment to the night clerk and continues on. Her office waits at the far end of the wing, tucked between records and diagnostics. It's a modest space lined with paperbacks, clinical journals, and a dying pothos plant she keeps forgetting to water. Meera flips on the light, sets her bag down with a gentle thud, and lets her body settle into the creaking chair that always lists slightly to the left. She doesn't open her laptop right away. She stares at the blank notepad on her desk and exhales. The silence is different here. It doesn't carry the hush of forgotten stories like the forest did, but it offers a place to begin assembling what she's found.

The hum of the ceiling fan is barely audible over the rustle of papers as Meera sets down her field notes and pulls up the burial demographic data she compiled over the last five years. Dada Jalam's words cling to her like the dust of Chikhalgaon, quiet, persistent, undeniable. She hasn't paid close attention to burial methods before, at least not beyond their cultural classifications. Now, something compels her to look deeper.

She runs cross-references between the new anomaly data and every environmental variable she can quantify—precipitation, groundwater salinity, agricultural runoff, pesticide drift. Each overlay produces noise but no pattern. The spikes she sees in one region vanish in the next. If the cause were chemical or climatic, the map would have bled in gradients. Instead, it stutters—local, uneven, defiant of geography.

She turns next to the biological archives, checking for shared ancestry among the affected families, then runs virology screens through the national database. Nothing holds. No common exposure, no pathogen, no genetic inheritance strong enough to explain the spread. The absence of connection leaves her uneasy; systems rarely fail this quietly, or this precisely. It feels less like a coincidence and more like something missing from the equations altogether.

As the hours pass, patterns emerge and the logic begins to unravel. The patterns show strong enough correlations to draw a pause, even if they don't point to causality directly. Villages with higher rates of sealed interment and imported concrete burial vaults show a sharper rise in birth anomalies over time. The trends aren't uniform, but they lean heavily in one direction. Sealed interment was meant to protect the living from the dead. Layers of concrete and regulation were added with the intent to quiet what lay beneath. By every standard model, nothing from those burial sites should touch the living ecosystem. And yet, their absence now appears to be the problem. It makes no sense.

Her pen moves quickly across the page now, forming loops and arrows and questions. What if transgenerational genetic drift wasn't just biochemical? What if the ecological feedback loop, that physical, microbial, material reintegration of organic memory is part of the genome's long-term stability? What if, by sealing the dead away from the soil, they're severing a generational nutrient stream they never even knew existed?

Meera sits back, unsure. Is she oversimplifying the data? Is she letting the poetry of Dada Jalam's memory carry her too far from empirical footing? The implications of what she's observing feel impossibly large and dangerously close to metaphor. Could something as ordinary as burial practices, which are changed by modernization and infrastructure, truly have this kind of generational biological impact? Is she seeing real patterns, or chasing stories dressed up as science?

She closes her eyes and debates the merits of holding the research a while longer. Maybe it needs refinement. More peer input. Maybe she's just captivated by the beauty and clarity of an idea that echoes the stillness she felt in the burial forest.

But part of her knows what the other part resists. The data is real. The trends are consistent. Even if the mechanism is still obscure, the signal in the noise is strong enough to warrant a deeper look, by more eyes than hers.

She opens a new document and begins writing her call for collaboration, a note to the wider field. She shapes it like a question more than a claim: a short correspondence describing the rise in congenital anomalies, the absence of clear environmental cause, the pattern she can't explain. The title came quickly: "Post-Mortem Genetic Cycling and Ecosystem Reintroduction in Humic Environments." What follows takes hours. She works late into the night, stacking correlations, citations, and speculative models. She's careful, cautious in tone, yet clear in message. She frames it as a hypothesis, a signal worth investigating.

By the time she hits save, she realizes the paper has grown dense. Technical. Maybe too esoteric to catch immediate interest. But it's honest. And it's hers. She submits it to *The Indian Journal of Public Health Research and Development*, unsure if anyone will read past the abstract, but resolves to find out.

Meera sits back, blinking at the screen. Then she highlights a line and rewrites it in her notebook:

Observed patterns suggest perceived absence may have a measurable biological correlate.

CHAPTER 7
THE SILENCE THAT FOLLOWS

Two years earlier.

A sterile hospital room, half-lit by flickering fluorescents, where Andrew sits not as a neurologist, not as a researcher, but as a father whose world has just narrowed to a single phrase.

Variant of Unknown Significance.

It begins here, with the silence that has followed that phrase. A silence so complete it feels surgical.

Moments ago, Juniper was diagnosed. Now, in the hospital's family room, Andrew sinks into the stiffest chair, the kind designed for waiting more than for rest. His elbows press into his thighs, his hands lock loosely between his knees, and his shoulders curve inward as if protecting something fragile inside his chest. The green paint on the walls pretends to be calm but only conjures memories of surgical drapes and anxious hours spent on call. Above him, the ceiling hums under fluorescent lights that turn every surface a shade too pale.

He's been in rooms like this for most of his adult life. Some were clinical, some were tragic, but he's never been here as a parent. This shift knocks the breath from his lungs in quiet, relentless waves.

The scent of antiseptic clings to his clothes like a second skin. His hands tremble. He doesn't feel fear. It's the absence of action, from the unbearable stillness of having nothing to fix.

Sonia appears in the doorway with Junie's hand curled loosely in hers, their footsteps soft against the tile. Junie's head droops, her small body sluggish with exhaustion. One of her sleeves is damp. She splashed water at the sink, and Sonia didn't bother to change her. The girl's plush giraffe peeks from the crook of her arm, clutched tight in the way children hold the things they understand when the world around them doesn't make sense.

Andrew straightens as they enter, trying to smooth his expression into something neutral. Not clinical, not panicked. Just present. Sonia meets his eyes for only a second before turning back to Junie and kneeling to zip her jacket.

"She's wiped," Sonia murmurs, her voice calm and tired. "I told her we'd go straight home. I think she's holding it together just to prove she's fine."

Junie turns toward him, eyes glassy. "Can I have toast at home?" she asks quietly.

Andrew nods. "Of course. With jelly, if you want."

She nods once, satisfied, and rests her head against her mother's hip.

Sonia stands and smooths Junie's hair. Her movements are practiced, gentle, and efficient, like someone who's performed this act too many times. "She doesn't really understand what the doctor said," Sonia adds quietly. "Which is a small blessing, I guess."

Andrew stands but doesn't move toward them. He wants to hold Junie, but something in him hesitates. His hands feel heavy, unsure. He shakes them, trying to break free. The doctor in him is still parsing the language from the consult, replaying every word.

Sonia senses it.

"I'll take her," she says kindly. "She needs sleep. You need to sit."

He wants to argue. Wants to follow. Instead, he just nods.

"I'll text you when we're home," she adds, adjusting Junie's backpack.

"Thank you," Andrew offers softly.

Sonia turns to go. Junie waves with her giraffe. The door clicks shut behind them, and the silence returns, denser than before, pressed in by everything they didn't say.

Andrew remains standing, hands still at his sides, jaw tight. He exhales, but the breath comes out unevenly. His eyes drift toward the window, though the view reveals nothing. It's just the faint reflection of fluorescent light bouncing off the glass.

The silence presses in again. This time it carries voices.

He replays the consultation; every word etched into the folds of his memory. The exam room smelled like rubber hoses and too much hand sanitizer. He and Sonia sat side by side, knees touching, hands laced tightly together between them. Her grip was steady. His was damp. Across from them sat the pediatric neurologist. Andrew couldn't even remember her name. She adjusted her glasses and spoke with practiced precision, her voice careful, each word polished from too many repetitions.

"Juniper's development falls into the range of neurodevelopmental delay," she said, eyes flicking between their charts and their faces. "Her symptoms suggest a mild global delay. Speech, motor planning, and social transitions. Nothing extreme. Although consistent."

Andrew's throat went dry. He gave the smallest nod; the one doctors give when they understand the meaning beneath the words.

The neurologist continued, flipping a page. "We ran the full genetic panel. There is a variant present on chromosome seven. It's classified as a variant of unknown significance."

There it was. The phrase that's followed him ever since. Variant of unknown significance. A phrase meant to sound technical and neutral. But to Andrew, it echoed with absence. A diagnosis without a direction. A mystery wrapped in science.

"This region overlaps with what we typically associate with Williams syndrome," the neurologist said, her tone neutral and cautious. "Juniper's presentation, however, is atypical. She lacks some of the hallmark facial features and vascular complications we often see. It's possible this is a mild or partial expression, or even a related but distinct variant."

Andrew has heard of Williams. He'd studied its cognitive signatures, its unusual social behaviors. He knew the textbook features: the delicate facial structure, the musicality of speech, the unguarded warmth, but the name carried a quiet sorrow he'd never felt until now. None of it prepared him for hearing it spoken in reference to his own child.

"No immediate intervention is necessary at this time," she added, gently. "Therapies may help with motor coordination and communication, but there's no treatment for the genetic finding. It's still being studied. What matters most is her environment. Stability. Support. Structured encouragement."

Andrew remembers nodding again, but he didn't hear the rest. Just the hum of fluorescent lights and the blood rushing in his ears.

Sonia asked the right questions. She asked about therapy referrals, timelines, and support systems. Her voice was calm; her questions were clear. Andrew barely spoke.

Because he already knew. This wasn't something he could solve in a lab or scrub away in surgery. There was no clear path forward. No protocol. Only unknowns.

It started with little things. Junie's sentences formed more slowly than those of other children. Her fine motor skills lagged just enough to be noticed, nothing dramatic. Transitions threw her. Morning routines, bedtime, shifting from one room to another. They could unravel her day. Sonia saw it first, of course. She was a teacher. She was trained to notice early signs. Trained to listen beneath the noise. One night, long after Junie had gone to bed, Sonia looked across the dinner table and said, gently, "I think we should talk to someone. It might be nothing, but I'm seeing things that don't feel quite right."

Andrew resisted at first. Junie was bright. Curious. Her imagination was wild and gorgeous. Sure, she was different, but wasn't that what made her remarkable? Still, Sonia's words settled in his chest like fog, slowly thickening until he could no longer dismiss them. When Junie's kindergarten teacher echoed the same concern, and then their pediatrician, he pivoted from denial to inquiry.

Andrew snaps back to the present moment, back in the hospital. He stands alone in the waiting room, long after Sonia and Junie left for home. The room didn't change, but the stillness around him feels heavier, denser with everything unspoken. He lowers himself slowly into the chair again, his body tense, back rigid, as if slumping would loosen the grip he was trying to maintain.

Before him lay the scan printouts. EEG results. Developmental benchmarks. Copies of the genetic workup. He spreads them across the small coffee table, stacking and re-stacking as though order could somehow bring clarity. The data doesn't answer back. It just stares.

He traces one of Junie's EEG graphs with his fingertip. The spikes weren't obvious. No sharp indicators. No neon warning signs. But there's something in the rhythm that feels off. Asymmetrical. Delayed. Too smooth where there should be noise, too jittery where there should be calm. He's seen patterns like this before. Fragments in other children, usually buried deep in a file, marked for observation, where no follow-up was performed.

Sonia's voice from earlier floats into the silence: "This is your daughter, not a patient."

He knows that, but he also knows what he saw. More than what's written on the page, more than the data alone. It's what the data doesn't say. It's the absence that unnerves him. The clean family history. The clean metabolic panel. The clean prenatal chart. Too clean. He flips pages looking for something—anything—to anchor the narrative, to explain the gap.

Maybe it's just a fluke. Maybe this is exactly what the neurologist said. An anomaly. A partial expression. Williams syndrome, but faint. Blurred at the edges. Perhaps the missing features are simply a matter of genetic chance.

Except, what if they're not?

He closes the chart and exhales sharply, blinking into the buzzing overhead light. He suddenly remembers something. A patient from years ago. A boy with rhythmic tremors and language delay. No diagnosis. Just gaps. Gaps in development. Gaps in inheritance. A VUS on chromosome sixteen. At the time, Andrew dismissed it as inconclusive. Now, those inconclusive cases begin clustering in his mind.

One by one, they return. Children with borderline scans, strange regressions, clean genetics, but something clearly off. Children who don't fit. Who were never given answers. Whose parents were sent home with vague hope and vague fear.

Right then, he knows he won't sleep tonight. He can't.

He gathers the printouts in one hand, shrugs on his coat, and walks out into the cold parking lot. He doesn't remember getting into the car. Doesn't even remember turning the key. He just knows that, thirty minutes later, he's parked at the far end of their street, engine off, dome light dim as he rummages under the passenger seat.

His fingers brush the edge of a soft-cover notebook. Junie's. It's half-colored, a few pages filled with bright scribbles and traced letters. He flips to the back, where the pages are still clean. Then he pulls out a pen. The irony didn't escape him. Crayons and questions. Childhood and uncertainty.

He writes in bursts. Frantic, looping handwriting that crowds the pages. Not clinical notes. Not polished. This isn't for peer review or publication. This is for him. A containment space. A confession. A beginning.

The pen feels clumsy in his grip at first, too ordinary a tool for what he's trying to capture. The ink skips when he presses too hard, like his thoughts are moving faster than the page can absorb. He stops and exhales, and he starts again. Slower this time. More deliberate. He writes his daughter's initials at the top of the first page, marking the origin with the label "JT."

He flips back to earlier patients, ones who linger in his memory for no clinical reason. A boy with early-onset tics and exceptional musical memory. A girl whose verbal skills vanished over the span of three months. A toddler who laughed at shadows and couldn't be comforted by sound. None of them has a diagnosis. All have scans that are almost normal.

He writes each name in the margin, initials only. Just enough to jog his own memory. Then he adds the symptoms that refuse to sort themselves into categories. He draws little arrows between entries, writes side notes about family history, recurrence, blood work, and birth weight. He adds asterisks where the files had language like "unremarkable" or "no cause identified." Those phrases have always bothered him. It's what they leave out more than what they actually say.

On one page, he diagrams an EEG waveform from memory, pausing halfway to adjust it. He remembers how the waveform made him pause when he first saw it years ago. Now he sees it again in Junie's. They're not identical, but they're close enough to make his chest tighten.

He doesn't realize how long he's been writing until his hand cramps. The car's dark now, the dome light flickering to darkness. The glow from the streetlamp outside spills over the dashboard. He shifts his weight and immediately feels the ache in his knees. He hasn't moved for over an hour.

But on the seat beside him is the beginning of something new. A growing ledger of not-knowing. A record of conditions and contradictions. A list of questions that refuse to provide answers.

By the time he sets the pen down, the notebook holds more than a dozen entries. Rough, imprecise, but unmistakably alive. The pages give him something to hold onto. The act of writing was cathartic. The questions are still questions. The anomalies are still unresolved. And yet, now at least, they're named. Collected. Traced.

He sits in the quiet car, his breath fogging faintly against the windows, and he stares at the closed notebook on the passenger seat. It feels a bit like a breakthrough. More than that, it feels like an invocation. He doesn't know what he's chasing yet, but it has weight. Shape. Direction. And it begins here.

In the following weeks, he returns to the notebook at odd hours. After rounds, before breakfast, and late at night when Sonia and Junie are asleep and the house is quiet. The pages fill in uneven bursts with ink smudges where he's nodded off mid-thought, diagrams with arrows that trail into the margins, and questions left hanging like unfinished prayers. Some nights, he feels the work pulling him under, the same cases circling in his mind until he can almost hear them breathing.

He begins color-coding symptom clusters. Mapping recurrence. He develops shorthand: VU for variant unknown, INH for inheritance irregularity, SEP for symptom expression plateau. He draws connections between seemingly unrelated cases. Between a toddler in Boston with mild hypotonia and an adolescent in New Zealand with identical speech irregularities. Between family trees that look unrelated until their branches begin to twist toward one another.

Patterns begin to emerge, fragile at first, like constellations glimpsed through fog. The more he catalogs, the more certain he becomes that something is slipping. Slowly, what begins as unanswered questions starts to cohere. Each time he revisits a case file, the same thought creeps in: something old appears to be fading.

The cases don't reveal a new disease, but they suggest a kind of genomic erosion. A softening of expression across generations. He writes that phrase down and circles it twice, then stares at it until the ink bleeds through the page. These aren't deletions. Not mutations. A missing robustness. Like a map printed with less ink each time. Something once present but now fading.

He revisits environmental factors. He blames the environment at first. Pollutants. Stress hormones. Chemical exposure. He overlays timelines of industrial expansion, dietary shifts, climate metrics, even population density curves. Each dataset promises clarity, then dissolves. But the more he searches, the less the timelines match. The less the exposure maps explain. The less the data resolves.

He stares at the curves and begins to see absence instead of presence. Then he wonders, what if it's not the environment acting on us, but something else? Something that's missing. A retreat. A quiet erasure.

One night, he wakes at the kitchen table, pen still in hand, a single unfinished thought whispering through his exhaustion. He pauses, the question forming before he can stop it. What if the blueprint itself is fading? He grips the pen tighter, afraid that writing it down will make it real. Then he catches himself and rephrases it on paper:

Observation: potential attenuation in baseline genomic expression; pattern degradation suspected.

The notebook closes with a soft thud. Outside, the first hint of dawn spills across the blinds. The Archive grows. Slowly. Quietly. With purpose. Each entry, each hypothesis, becomes less about solving a mystery and more about bearing witness to what may already be slipping away.

And Junie? She grows, too. Brilliant, unpredictable, and wholly herself. Andrew never stops being her father. Still, he never stops being a scientist either. Even as he plays Legos with her on the carpet or watches her sort jellybeans by color and narrate a plush-toy banquet, the patterns hum in the back of his mind.

On one particular rainy Thursday night, the house smells like cinnamon toast and anchovies. Junie's chosen dinner after rejecting everything else in the fridge. Andrew kneels beside her at the dining table, helping her realign the rainbow tiles of her plastic mosaic. She's humming tunelessly, lost in the task, her tongue poking out between her teeth as she concentrates.

"Green next?" Andrew asks.

"No," Junie says confidently. "That's a sky spot. It has to be blue."

He nods, corrected. "Obviously."

She giggles and presses the tile into place.

In the next room, Sonia reads a paper on her tablet, curled on the couch with a throw blanket wrapped around her legs. Her hair is up, damp from the quick shower she managed after getting home late from school conferences. She watches the scene over the rim of her mug. Andrew and Junie hunched like co-conspirators over a masterpiece that would later be forgotten on the floor.

Once the oven chimes that dinner is ready, they all move to the kitchen. They eat late, all three at the kitchen island. Junie narrates her day in winding spirals. Something about a squirrel in the school court-yard, a mystery involving a missing crayon, and a bold declaration that carrots make terrible currency for playground trade. Sonia listens with practiced grace, responding in the same voice she uses with her most imaginative students. Curious, engaged, and grounded. Andrew mostly listens too, his mind flickering between the kitchen's soft light and the fragments of questions still echoing from the Archive.

At the end of the evening, after Junie's tucked in and the giraffe positioned just right on the pillow and her lamp glowing lavender through a star-shaped bulb, Andrew finds Sonia folding laundry in their bedroom. He offers to help. They don't talk much at first, just move in rhythm, the kind of sync only built over years of shared space.

Eventually, Sonia says, "She used the word 'hypothesis' today."

Andrew glances up. "She did?"

"She said her hypothesis was that marshmallows would melt in her lunchbox if it stayed in the sun too long."

He smiles, folding a T-shirt. "She's going to be a scientist."

"She gets it from you."

"She gets her persistence from you."

Sonia laughs. "And the glitter."

They stand quietly for a moment, then Sonia adds, "She's doing okay, you know."

"I know," Andrew agrees. And he does. Yet, he also feels the pull. The need to understand why Junie's path bent differently from others.

Later, Sonia climbs into bed with a new book with a bright cover and a hopeful title. Andrew hesitates in the doorway to his office. She notices.

"Still thinking?"

He nods. "Just want to jot down a few things before I forget. A case from residency. Something it's connecting to."

She doesn't press. "Don't stay up too late."

"I won't," he says.

She's already turning the page as he closes the door.

It isn't long after that night, months after Junie's diagnosis, that Sonia finds the notebook. She sets it gently on Andrew's desk and states, "Whatever you're chasing, don't forget to live in the meantime."

He doesn't forget. He also doesn't stop.

Because in the data, in the silence, in the growing pages of the Archive, he sees something forming. A whisper of a theory. A shape. The outline of a truth that science hasn't made room for.

For the first time since that night in the hospital family room, Andrew doesn't feel helpless.

He feels awake.

CHAPTER 8
FIRST CONTACT

Andrew sits hunched over his desk in the solitude of his home office, a halo of dim light illuminating a semicircle of printouts and sticky notes. The room smells faintly of wood and dust. Junie is asleep upstairs, and Sonia went to bed long ago. The house is dim and still. Around him lay years of handwritten notes pulled from his personal vault of questions and unsolved threads. The margins are filled with frustrated scrawls, underlined symptoms, VUS codes, and timelines that spanned over a decade of pediatric neurology. Now, he is trying to stitch them together. To see whether the pattern is real, and perhaps to help make sense of what Junie is experiencing.

He compiles everything. Every patient entry with an unresolved marker, every EEG anomaly that defied classification. He cross-references geographic distribution with environmental exposure, plots developmental delays across regions, and highlights subtle behavioral regressions that were never included in official diagnoses. His charts pulse with color-coded highlights and annotated flags. They blanket the wall behind him and spill onto the floor, like a neurodevelopmental crime scene. And in the center of it all, on his screen, glows the first coherent synthesis he has ever attempted to write.

What emerges is a signal. The evidence points past a single syndrome or shared mutation. Instead, it whispers of erosion. A fading complexity across cases that have nothing in common, and yet, so much in common. Andrew doesn't see a disease. What he sees is a subtraction. Something missing. Something quiet. A trait unpassed.

The next morning, the hospital hums with its usual choreography of chirping phones and intercoms in between the hustle of doctors and nurses moving swiftly through the halls. Andrew's office door clicks once, then swings wider without a knock.

"Theo," Andrew says, glancing up from a stack of charts. "You look like you haven't slept."

"I haven't," Theo replies, dropping his bag into the corner chair. "You know that flash drive you gave me last week? I spent most of the night with it."

Andrew straightens a little. "And?"

Theo exhales, rubbing the bridge of his nose. "Been thinking about your absence theory. I had to let it sit for a few days, but it kept bugging me. I think you might be onto something. It just feels like it might be early."

Andrew tilts his head. "Meaning?"

"Meaning you're pointing to something real, but it doesn't have shape yet. The data seems rather quiet right now. Still, I ran another pass on your flagged cases. Cross-referenced them with our historical cohort data."

Andrew's pulse quickens. "And?"

"That's the thing," Theo says, pulling up a tablet. "What stood out wasn't what was there. It was what was missing. Consistently low expression levels on several developmental genes. Faint anomalies in methylation patterns that don't align with any known exposures. It's too aligned to ignore but inconsistent enough to call definitive."

Andrew's eyes flicker between the tablet and Theo's expression. "So not contamination?"

"No. Not unless every lab on three continents is making the same mistake." Theo scrolls through data overlays. "Here's the part that really got me. When we built a timeline of symptom onset and laid it over localized environmental data—soil composition, heat index, even urban development—we found weak correlations. Present, but not causal."

Andrew sits back, the idea forming even before Theo voices it.

"If we're seeing deactivation rather than damage," Theo continues, "then maybe we've been looking at the wrong thing all along."

For a moment, the room hums only with the distant intercom. Andrew studies him. "You're saying it might not be what's happening to the genome but what's disappearing from it."

Theo nods once. "Exactly. You're not crazy, Andrew. You might just be early."

Andrew lets out a small breath, the corners of his mouth twitching in what could almost be a smile. "You have no idea how good it is to hear someone else say that."

Theo shrugs. "Don't get sentimental on me, but it's worth cataloging what's present and missing. That's where we start."

Andrew turns to his monitor, already typing notes. "We'll need a refined comparative analysis to look closer at the methylation gaps, see if they track through heritability markers."

"I can do that," Theo says. "And soil exposure data against maternal age cohorts?"

Andrew nods. "Exactly."

Theo grins, a flash of mischief cutting through his fatigue. "You realize this means I'm signing up for sleepless nights again."

"Good," Andrew says, without looking up. "I'd hate to be the only one."

For the first time in months, he feels something move forward inside him. Propulsion. Theo's skepticism is the best kind of validation. Someone with rigor saw the same gaps, the same faint symmetry, and still wanted to look closer.

He wants more than support now. He wants Theo to test the boundaries of the idea, to try and disprove it, to stress the logic until only what is sound remains. Because if the gaps hold, if the data points to absence rather than an anomaly, then this might be more than theory. It might be a foundation for something new.

Standing up, Andrew paces once around the room, then sits again with a renewed sense of purpose. If Theo sees it, then maybe others will as well. And maybe, just maybe, he is on the edge of something worth pursuing aloud.

He isn't alone.

Over the following week, the meetings become routine, beginning early in Andrew's office or ending late in Theo's data lab. Their screens glow with side-by-side datasets: patient histories, environmental charts, molecular readouts.

Theo gestures toward a heatmap on his monitor. "This is the subset you flagged. The cases with partial overlap in onset age. I re-ran the comparative analysis using our internal normalization algorithm. It tightened the variance, but the outliers remain."

Andrew leans over, squinting at the gradient scale. "Outliers by what measure?"

"Expression amplitude," Theo offers. "See here. The regions in blue should correlate to minimal deviation, but these patches shift into orange without any clear environmental factor."

Andrew nods slowly. "Could that be a calibration error?"

Theo shakes his head. "Already checked. Different instruments, same skew."

Andrew starts sketching a quick overlay on the whiteboard. "Then let's map them geographically. Maybe there's a local variance we're not accounting for, like climate, population density, something hidden in the soil or water index."

Theo joins him at the board. "You're assuming proximity still matters," he says.

"Until it doesn't," Andrew replies, drawing overlapping circles that connect the clusters. "Let's see what holds when we compare it to the developmental markers."

For a while, the only sound is the scratch of markers and the faint hum of the server rack. Theo switches to his tablet, sketching a comparative heatmap as Andrew dictates coordinates. The patterns begin to emerge—subtle, incomplete, but suggestive.

Theo studies the result. "Strange symmetry," he murmurs.

Andrew exhales, resting his hand on the back of a chair. "It's something we haven't learned to ask yet."

Theo grins faintly. "That's your specialty, isn't it?"

"Questions?"

"No," Theo says, tapping the heatmap. "Asking them before the rest of us are ready."

Andrew doesn't answer, but a quiet satisfaction settles between them. What began as a solitary curiosity is becoming a shared pursuit. They are two minds circling the same puzzle from opposite ends.

Theo never misses a chance at levity, and one morning greets Andrew at the Starbucks across from the hospital. It is their unspoken neutral ground. A place that removes them from pagers and corridor traffic, where the scent of roasted beans cuts through the haze of clinical procedures.

Theo slides into their usual table by the window, waving a printout above his head like he is auctioning off a rare artifact. In his other hand, he balances a grande cold brew and a protein bar. His ID badge hangs loose around his neck, flipped backward as usual.

"Okay, I admit it, you were right about that methylation cluster," he says, his grin pulling wide. "But if this ends with me presenting at a paranormal genetics conference, I'm blaming you."

"So, you're good with rewriting our understanding of pediatric inheritance but throw in one unexplained absence and you're out?" Andrew snaps back.

"Exactly," Theo deadpans. "Next thing I know, you'll be quoting crop circle statistics."

They trade barbs as naturally as they trade data. Andrew teases Theo about his rainbow-colored spreadsheets. "You realize Excel isn't a mood ring, right?" with Theo shooting back about Andrew's hyper-labeled archive folders, "You've got footnotes on your footnotes. I'm considering an intervention."

Yet behind the jokes lies something more serious, a growing possibility.

Theo brings in historical cohorts and genomic profiles from his department's database, and Andrew layers in developmental timelines and unpublished EEG records from the Archive. They annotate spreadsheets, redline early drafts, and even toy with building a shared model for mapping genetic erosion across age brackets. They debate over null hypotheses, challenge each other's assumptions, and refine their parameters with the intensity of a research team on the edge of something vital.

At Theo's urging, Andrew begins drafting what the medical world would call a perspective brief. A format somewhere between editorial and formal publication. The task does not come easily. For three nights in a row, he writes and deletes the opening paragraph, unsure how bold is too bold or how subtle is too safe. Each word feels like a gamble. Push too far, and he risks dismissal; hedge too much, and he loses meaning.

He thinks about Junie. About her quiet questions and her collection of wind chimes, each one chosen for its tone. She hangs them by mood. Bright ones for happy mornings, low tones for quiet afternoons. About how she once asked why no two chimes made the same sound, and whether that meant they each had a secret name. He thinks about the medical charts that still fail to name what she carries in her genes. He thinks about the families of other children who never had someone take a second look. Andrew considers it a moral responsibility.

At times, Andrew feels the pull of old colleagues' warnings. "Stick to the data," they used to say. "Don't court speculation." Then he also hears Theo's voice, challenging and electric: "Maybe we've been looking at the wrong thing all along."

In the margins of his draft, Andrew scribbles fragments of truth he can't fit into the manuscript. Lines like "What if absence is the signal?" and "Can degradation be its own fingerprint?"

Eventually, he settles on a tone. Neutral, rigorous, open-ended. He doesn't want to make claims; he wants to make space. A crack in the wall wide enough for light to pass through. He writes cautiously, every word chosen with care. He strips emotion from the language and lets the data speak. He references studies on environmental epigenetics, prenatal exposure, and developmental drift. He frames his findings as an observational anomaly cluster, not a discovery. But in the undercurrent, his intent is clear: someone needs to look deeper.

He reads over the closing paragraph again:

Preliminary analysis indicates recurring reductions in non-pathological gene expression across unrelated cohorts. No shared exposures identified. Environ-

mental factors insufficient to explain the magnitude or directionality of change. Patterns suggest a systemic attenuation in baseline expression rather than an external disruption. Additional data and peer input are requested before further interpretation.

The title was deliberately neutral: "Genetic Drift in Pediatric Neurodevelopmental Disorders." It captures the heart of the absence theory without making direct claims. He submits it to a mid-tier open-access pediatric neurology journal known for publishing exploratory work. It is a professional risk. If colleagues read too far between the lines, it could be dismissed as speculative. Stepping past that fear, Andrew is done waiting for permission. He doesn't need the paper to be definitive. He needs to know if anyone else sees what he sees.

Two weeks later, an email pops into his inbox.

The subject line: *Overlap in anomaly clusters? Response to your recent article.*

The sender: Dr. Meera Rao.

Andrew's pulse quickens. He pushes his chair back, crosses the room, and pulls the Archive from his satchel. It opens right to the page. He had underlined her name and copied the quote that haunted him ever since: "Human remains interred in sterile, sealed environments fail to reintegrate genetic material into the local biome. Over successive generations, communities with high embalming and coffin-seal rates may inadvertently disrupt transgenerational genomic replenishment."

He wrote her name in the margin, followed by a question mark and a single word: *possible?*

Several weeks ago, Andrew came across that article, quietly published in a regional open-access environmental health journal. At the time, he thought the line was poetic. Speculative, maybe. Now, it reads like the missing half of a sentence he started to write.

He immediately clicks the email, his heart picking up pace. The message is concise yet rich with insight. Meera introduces herself as a clinical researcher working with congenital defect data in rural India. She came across his article through a shared search alert on pediatric neurodevelopmental delay. Her tone is professional, her language precise, and threaded through her sentences is a familiar urgency.

She references two of his anomaly groupings, then highlights several parallel cases from her own fieldwork. Her approach is markedly different. She is approaching the issue from the perspective of environmental and population health, rather than neurology. Her tools are statistical software and village interviews. Still, the findings are specific and startling.

She includes data from three distinct rural communities bordering the sacred burial forest. In each, she tracks a rising trend of congenital anomalies over the past several decades, controlling for maternal age, birth order, and access to prenatal care. In one village, the rate of reported neural tube defects has doubled in seven years. In other cases, cardiac irregularities in newborns have clustered around families with no identifiable genetic predisposition. She includes soil samples, noting elevated levels of trace preservatives and heavy metals in areas near modernized burial plots. Meera observes a correlation between the shift in burial customs. Specifically, the transition from traditional open-air or biodegradable methods to cement-sealed interment and the resulting disruptions in local microbial biodiversity. She postulates that these microbiome changes could influence prenatal development through environmental exposure, although she was careful not to overstate the connection.

Her manuscript poses no definitive cause. However, it points to a pattern. One with biological plausibility and sufficient nuance to merit further investigation.

Andrew read it once. Then again. Then a third time, slower.

She isn't saying the same thing as him, but she's asking the same question.

Andrew replies that same night, heart pounding as he types. The data from Meera's manuscript pulses in his mind. Not the whole of it, just a particular thread. The recurring anomalies in regions of high-density sealed burials. One dataset in particular stands out. A village where anomalies begin to appear within two generations after a shift to structured interments.

He can't stop thinking about the parallels. It's not just geographic. It's not just developmental. It's temporal. As if something changes in the years that follow death. Accumulating like sediment in the soil.

His breath catches at the thought. He's terrified by the implication that human ritual, sacred and protective, might have an unintended echo. He's also electrified. For the first time, someone else sees it too. And she isn't backing away. She's leaning in.

His message is longer than hers, filled with gratitude and curiosity. He references the anomaly spikes in her community study and overlays them against his own patient registry, pointing out three children from Texas, Arizona, and New Mexico who presented with near-identical EEG irregularities and developmental gaps during the same seasonal windows Meera identified for anomaly spikes in Maharashtra.

He highlights a shared age-of-onset curve that clusters around eighteen to twenty-four months, a period when critical neurodevelopment typically accelerates. He matches that to her own spike in reported sensory integration issues in the Bhira region. He includes anonymized case notes, including one particularly complex case with persistent subcortical hyperactivity and no identifiable genetic cause.

He asks for her interpretation of a VUS flag that has appeared in two siblings. One was diagnosed with generalized hypotonia, and the other with a speech delay and mild tremors. The same variant has appeared in one of the region-adjacent cases from her manuscript.

Then, after reviewing the overlapping data one more time, he closes with a line he didn't expect to write:

I think we're looking at two sides of the same coin.

For a moment, Andrew sits back and lets the words linger on the screen. It feels like a pivot point. One of those rare moments in research when the fog shifts just enough to suggest the shape of a path ahead. He doesn't need to convince Meera. She's already running her own thread through the same knot.

Over time, what starts as formal emails soon evolves into deeper exchanges. One night, after a dense chain of statistical comparisons, Meera adds a line at the end of her message. "Sometimes I wonder if we're chasing the echo of something sacred and forgotten but still present." The words linger longer than Andrew expects.

From there, the rhythm of their communication begins to shift. They still speak in code and ratios, yes, but also in glimpses of their lives. Field stories. Family quirks. Moments of doubt. The data remains at the center, and around it, something human grows.

Over the next two weeks, they send messages almost daily. They dissect statistical patterns, question each other's assumptions, and argue over possible sources of bias. They share graphs and anecdotes, stray observations and hunches. Sometimes they pause to check each other's enthusiasm. Is this real, or are they seeing meaning where there is none? Through the questioning and moments of doubt, their correspondence never slows.

By the end of the second week, their conversations outgrew the limits of email. They begin holding regular video consults, syncing across time zones as best they can. Andrew often starts his day early in Austin to sync up with Meera's late afternoon. Meera joining from her office in Hyderabad, surrounded by stacks of field reports and the occasional rustle of monsoon winds through the cracked window.

During these sessions, they share screens, annotate real-time data, and adjust hypothesis parameters with the ease of colleagues who have worked together for years. Andrew watches Meera map rural cluster trends with remarkable speed, her fieldwork sharpened by instinct and repetition, while Meera marvels at the precision of Andrew's clinical timelines and the structure of his logic. He annotates symptom progressions with an eye for both pattern and story.

Sometimes Junie peeks in behind her father, clutching a stuffed animal or holding a glass of milk, drawn by the flicker of the screen and the soft rhythm of her father's voice. She doesn't always speak, but her presence grounds the moment. Meera always pauses to greet her, sometimes switching briefly into a lighter tone. On one occasion, Junie points to Meera's window on the screen and asks, "Who's that?"

"That's Dr. Meera. She's my science friend," Andrew replies.

"She looks nice," Junie whispers, as if Meera might hear her.

"Thank you, Junie," Meera says kindly. "I hear you're the scientist in your house."

Junie puffs her chest slightly. "I made a volcano last week. It exploded on purpose."

Meera laughs. "Then you're already ahead of most of us."

Junie grins and then whispers to her dad, "Tell your friend she should add glitter when she builds her volcano."

Andrew shook his head with a smile. "Tough crowd."

Those brief interludes remind Andrew why he's chasing the data in the first place. He isn't just decoding cases; he's decoding his own daughter. Yet, in those fleeting moments of joy and connection, he can see that Junie is not a problem to solve. She is a wonder to protect. Meera seems to understand that without it ever being said aloud.

Their language grows more fluid with each video call. Technical exchanges become layered with trust. What began as correspondence becomes collaboration. Perhaps something more foundational. They aren't just comparing notes anymore. They are building a framework for understanding something neither has been able to name on their own.

Andrew finds her sharp, open, and unafraid to challenge his thinking. During one late-night consult, she pushes back on his assumption that symptom onset timing alone could serve as a proxy for environmental exposure. "That kind of correlation," she says, "needs context from maternal history, from regional soil cycles. Otherwise, it's just another floating variable."

Andrew bristles for a moment, his instinct to defend rising before he recognizes her point. He exhales, adjusts the timeline, and concedes. "You're right. I was oversimplifying."

It isn't contentious. It's clarifying. Meera challenges him to refine his observation, and he finds the friction invigorating.

Meera finds him precise, grounded, but willing to stretch into the unknown. Their disciplines rarely intersect in academic circles, but in the space between their inboxes, a collaboration took root.

They're still working on the theory, but in the meantime, they have questions that they keep asking.

What aren't we seeing?

Why does it keep repeating?

CHAPTER 9
GHOST GENOME

A montage of discovery unfolds with quiet deliberation, each moment purposeful and exacting. It begins with spreadsheets open across two time zones, video calls scribbled with digital annotations, and virtual whiteboards filled with overlapping datasets. EEG scans flicker on one screen while soil charts render slowly on another. Meera drags her cursor across a map of microbial density in rural Maharashtra, and Andrew sketches a corresponding trend on his touchscreen tablet, circling areas that mimic neural irregularities. Sometimes, they speak in bursts. Half-sentences. Shorthand. The kind of fluent crosstalk that only emerges when two minds start aligning.

One evening, after Meera highlights an anomaly she can't fully decode, Andrew pushes back against his chair and says, "I think it's time we bring in Theo."

"Theo Manning?" she asks.

"Yes. He's a genomic systems guy. Bit of a cynic, but he sees patterns most people miss. He can run batch queries and expression overlays in his sleep."

Meera raises an eyebrow, intrigued. "He won't laugh us out of the room?"

Andrew smiles. "He might stay, and if he does, we'll know we're onto something real."

Theo's first call with them is, in his words, "a cross between a TED Talk and a conspiracy podcast." He logs in wearing a wrinkled hoodie and a mug that says, "Trust No One," clearly bracing for entertainment rather than enlightenment. There's a poster on the wall behind him that looks like a medical advertisement that reads, "I peer review people now."

The connections feel quiet at first. Then, about ten minutes in, his posture shifts. His eyebrows rise slightly as Meera explains the strange overlap in congenital anomalies and regional burial customs. He leans forward when Andrew pulls up an EEG overlay that defies classification.

"Wait," Theo interrupts, frowning. "Run that last set again. What's the control group look like?"

Andrew flicks through slides, narrating in clipped, careful language. Theo stops him again, pointing. "There. That's not noise. That's a shadow pattern. You don't see it often unless you're looking at epigenetic regression curves."

He sits back, rubbing the bridge of his nose. "Okay, I came for the show. But I'm staying for the math."

Theo expected only a polite skim, but something about their persistence and the weird elegance of the anomalous patterns holds his curiosity. He's spent most of his career in cancer genomics, crunching datasets that promise too much and deliver too little. He once left a high-profile lab after blowing the whistle on statistical manipulation in a major paper. Since then, he has built a reputation as a skeptic with a sharp algorithmic mind and a low tolerance for scientific melodrama.

His involvement carries weight and arrives with sincerity. He listens as Meera describes overlapping patterns in congenital anomalies tied to burial practices and microbial shifts, and Andrew lays out EEG signatures that defy known classification.

"So, let me get this straight," Theo says, spinning slowly in his desk chair. "You two think dirt might be messing with our DNA? Should I be composting more aggressively?"

Andrew chuckles. "We're saying the inheritance model might be incomplete. There's a suppression pattern forming. We think environmental integration, or the lack of it, might be a missing variable."

"And you want me to bless it with some algorithmic fairy dust," Theo replies, mock solemn. "Well, I'm in. But only if I get naming rights when this turns into the next scientific scandal."

From that point forward, Andrew, Meera, and Theo develop a shared rhythm. Their harmony, however, develops gradually. Early on, they stumble over each other's language. Andrew's clinical shorthand frustrates Theo, who prefers clean variable names and reproducible code. Meera speaks in patterns and public health metaphors, which Theo calls "beautifully imprecise." One call ends in silence after a heated back-and-forth over a mismatched soil sample, and Andrew sends a long Slack message trying to smooth it over.

A shift begins when Meera walks Theo through her classification logic using a color-coded spreadsheet and a story about two neighboring villages with opposite birth outcomes. Theo doesn't interrupt but instead rewrites her algorithm in real time and adds a note: "Your metaphor was better. But here's the math version."

By the following week, their jargon begins to overlap. Theo adjusts his language to accommodate Meera's regional exposure layers, and Andrew starts tagging EEG cases with Theo's clustering labels. A rhythm forms gradually, each movement adding to a growing cadence. They move from parallel solvers to something more like an ensemble, each voice distinct, but resonant. Each brings a different lens. Andrew's grounded in neurology and lived experience; Meera's rooted in epidemiology and environmental systems; and Theo, ever the molecular architect, turns genomic fog into legible models. Even though their languages differ, they begin to harmonize over time.

Andrew's Archive sets the tone. His data whispers of children born with absences, gaps where complexity should have flourished, distinct from known syndromes. Variants appear inconclusive on paper but recur in ways no model can explain. No trauma. No environmental exposure. No clear lines. Just children with missing complexity. Subtle neurological gaps that mimic known disorders but don't follow the rules.

Meera overlays his cases with regional environmental data from India.

Birth defect trends tied to burial customs and shifts in microbial density around sacred forest grounds. She sees the same shape in her soil charts that Andrew sees in EEG spikes. Distinct in their content, aligned in their trajectory. A slope instead of a spike. Drift instead of rupture.

Andrew studies the merged plot. The shapes aren't just similar—they feel sequential, as if her anomalies mark the body's first missed instructions and his recordings capture the echoes of those same instructions fading in the brain.

"What if it's all one process," he says quietly. "Early silence leaves fingerprints on the body. Later silence settles in the mind."

Meera doesn't answer right away, but the look she gives him says she's already thought it.

Theo brings method to the madness. He builds a recursive model that tracks expression slippage, focusing on reductions rather than deletions. He parses out silent markers, epigenetic changes with no apparent cause, and maps them over time. In several cases, the same "silent genes" flicker across families in both hemispheres. These genes aren't switched off or mutated; they remain present in form while subdued in their expression.

"If the silencing happens in the first weeks," Theo says, drawing a flat line through the earliest phase of his graph, "you get physical malformation potentially in organs or limbs, the visible stuff. If it happens later, when the cortex is wiring, you may get neural quiet. Different timing, same silence."

Andrew zooms in on the curve, tracing it on the screen with his finger. "That same drop at 200 hertz is identical to what we saw in the tissue samples," he says.

Meera leans closer, her camera feed flickering in the corner of his monitor. "You're right. The same pattern etched in bone is showing up in EEG data now. That can't be a coincidence."

Across the shared drive, Theo uploads a new dataset. "Hold on," he says. "These three cases from Chile are clean. No microbial anomalies, no burial irregularities, nothing."

"That doesn't make sense," Meera replies. "If the pattern's genuine, something should tie them together. Either contamination, or—"

"Not contamination," Theo interrupts. "The cluster's real. I double-checked the attenuation markers myself."

Andrew rubs his temple. "Let's not jump. Maybe the recordings were mislabeled."

Two days blur together as they trade redlines and recalibrated graphs across time zones. Theo curses at missing filters; Meera defends her parameters. "You're smoothing out real signal," she insists.

"And you're chasing noise," Theo fires back.

Andrew's voice cuts through, calm but firm. "Check the source files again. Line by line."

An hour later, Theo exhales sharply. "Found it."

Meera looks up. "Found what?"

"The hospital's metadata was wrong. These kids weren't from the city. They're from a farming region outside it. Landfills there just started using soil-capping protocols. That microbial data was excluded from our primary map."

Meera sits back, briefly silent. "So, the anomaly isn't random. It's geographical."

Andrew nods. "And it means the absence isn't spreading by chance."

Theo's message pings across the thread.

"Turns out I was wrong," he writes, "but only because I was partially right. My favorite kind."

Meera lets out a laugh. "Partial credit accepted."

Andrew smiles. "Let's make that a rule. No single variable gets the spotlight until it proves it can hold the stage."

"Fine," Theo replies. "Then what's our next act?"

"Boundaries," Meera says. "Before the curve means anything, we test where it breaks."

From her end, she reruns the soil assays, tweaking for runoff, pesticide drift, and the change in crop rotations. Andrew works through hospital data, cross-referencing case histories with housing records and maternal nutrition logs.

"I've ruled out industrial exposure, air quality, and metals," he says one morning, eyes fixed on the patient overlays. "None of it aligns."

Theo appears in the video window, arms folded. "You're telling me we're seeing absence, but if you don't prove there's no smoking gun buried in that dirt, figuratively or literally, I'm calling it noise."

Andrew chuckles. "You think I haven't looked for one?"

Meera rolls her eyes. "Fine. Challenge accepted." She uploads another dataset. "Here—geotagged environmental metrics. Nitrate levels, electro-magnetic exposure, groundwater flow."

Theo drags the files into his interface. "All right. Let's see what the map thinks." Lines of code flash across his screen as he overlays pediatric genomics with satellite imagery, plotting patient coordinates against power substations.

An hour later, he sits up straight. "Hold on. Southern Arizona just lit up."

"Same attenuation?" Meera asks.

"No," Theo says. "Different. This one's messy. There are abrupt fluctu-ations instead of fades."

Andrew frowns and pulls up the EEG file. The waveform jitters like a skipped heartbeat. "That's not noise," he murmurs. "It's oscillating."

Theo runs a comparison model against their standard attenuation curve. "Nope. This spike doesn't taper. It climbs and then plateaus. Almost like a hyperactive scaffold."

Meera squints at the environmental layer. "Could it be artificially enhanced? Maybe the area has undergone recent remediation?"

They pull zoning records and discover the site was part of a rewilding project. It was formerly overgrazed land, and now it's saturated with compost and biochar intended to restore topsoil and water retention. "So, we've got a localized biosphere bounce," Meera notes. "That could create a unique microbial bloom."

"But why the neurological shift?" Andrew presses. "Isn't this too fast for generational feedback?"

Theo's eyes narrow. "Unless it's not generational. Unless the change happens prenatally, in response to hyper-dense scaffolding. A kind of genomic surge."

A long silence follows.

"That would mean," Meera says slowly, "our curve isn't just a slope toward silence. It might have inflection points, moments where environmental pressure either suppresses or accelerates expression."

Andrew exhales. "Which means our model just got more complicated. And more real."

"Okay, explain this," he says, sharing his screen. "Same anomalies, but look, no burial data. No microbial disruption. The attenuation curve spikes instead of softening."

Meera frowns. "Could be a reporting error or incomplete records."

Andrew looks directly at his screen. "Maybe we're measuring the wrong environmental axis."

Theo opens another tab and cross-references prenatal health data, then filters by soil pH and carbon saturation. After a few quiet minutes of clicking, he says, "Found it. The surrounding region was artificially enriched after a wildfire. Massive fungal bloom. Mycorrhizal density nearly tripled. These kids were born right after that window."

Meera nods slowly. "So instead of absence, there's a spike in environmental scaffolding. The genome is overcompensating."

Theo smirks. "Even the anomalies have anomalies. Yet, it still fits. It reinforces the curve, just from the other side."

He paused, then added, "And then there's this one."

He opened another tab and dragged a scan onto the shared screen. A pediatric EEG file, overlaid with genetic markers. "Came from a contact of mine in Helsinki. A neurology fellow there flagged it during a longitudinal sleep study on Arctic Circle children."

Andrew squinted. "Finland?"

"Yep. The child was born in a rural village near a peat bog. They still practice natural burial there. No caskets and no embalming. Just cloth and soil. The region is nutrient-rich, but the burial customs are pre-industrial."

Meera leaned closer. "And the EEG?"

"The exact inverse of what we're seeing in the attenuation zones. Elevated coherence in the prefrontal cortex. Advanced language onset. And here's the kicker: low regional rates of developmental delay. Near-zero. More importantly, they're not over-diagnosing or underreporting. The health infrastructure there is solid."

Andrew tapped his pen. "So, no drift?"

"None. If anything, it's the opposite. An overexpression curve. When we mapped the methylation markers, they were denser than baseline. More than healthy. Enriched."

Meera shook her head slowly. "We've been chasing absence. But maybe there are places where presence persists. Places that never severed the biological feedback loop."

Theo frowned thoughtfully. "Still, it can't just be burial customs. If entombment were the whole story, we'd see sharper divergence everywhere modern burial dominates."

Meera nodded. "Maybe we would, if other variables weren't masking it. Urban soil composition, industrial runoff, and disrupted microbial networks each could dull the signal. In places like that village, the loop stays intact long enough to register."

"So, environmental interference," Andrew said, finishing the thought.

"Or suppression," Meera replied. "Something layered over the signal, blurring it."

Theo tilts his head. "Then why aren't we seeing the inverse where burial's sealed? Vaults, embalming, the whole industrial system—you'd expect stronger signal loss, maybe even pathology."

Meera shakes her head. "We are, just not in sharp relief. Most high-density nations mask it with the infrastructure of medical intervention, nutrition, and prenatal care. The drift hides inside the noise. Subtle shifts in methylation don't announce themselves as crises; they dilute over generations."

Andrew adds quietly, "It's the attenuation of inheritance itself versus the absence in every cell. Industrial life cushions the impact, but the silence still spreads."

Theo nods. "This kid's data reads like the genome was getting everything it asked for and more."

Andrew leaned back, quietly stunned. "The attenuation isn't universal. It's contextual. Ecological."

Theo chimes in, "Well, I'm not buying this unless we test for climate pressure," he says, squinting at a set of rising temperature anomalies.

"Already done," Meera replies, flipping to a comparison layer. "Temperature rise doesn't track. Nor does population density or urban sprawl. We ruled out pesticide correlation too. The timing and geography are off."

"What about the power lines?" Theo asks.

"Mapped," Andrew says. "We removed every case within a thousand meters of a high-voltage corridor. Patterns hold."

Andrew whiteboards the residual cases with color-coded markers, sketching patterns as Theo watches via video call. "Pull the top ten percent for clustering," Theo directs. "If it vanishes when we randomize, we toss it. If it gets louder, we dig deeper."

As the data begins to cohere, they feel a responsibility to challenge it. The pattern seems too clean, too consistent, almost suspiciously so.

Each morning begins with new findings. Meera reviews the heatmap annotations from the previous night, while Andrew opens fresh soil sequencing results that Theo flagged from his overnight batch. Their Slack thread scrolls endlessly with redlines, marginalia, algorithm tweaks, and flagged anomalies. Whiteboard snapshots ping across time zones, notes scrawled in marker: "Check methylation here," "Rerun cohort B," "Exclude samples near tertiary roads." What started as fragments now threads into something taut and strangely coherent. Somewhere between their uploads and revisions, the unnamed theory gains momentum and begins to speak for itself.

Without planning for it, the work often follows them into the hours when nothing productive should be happening.

Their shared Slack thread continues to evolve into a kind of running journal, filled with late-night theories, half-baked metaphors, and files uploaded at odd hours.

In one thread, Meera attached a new soil sequencing result that showed microfauna depletion in a recently cemented graveyard on the outskirts of Pune. Theo chimed in with a GIF of a washing machine in flames captioned, "Me running a heatmap cluster before caffeine." It was immediately followed by a serious annotation, "Check lateral methylation dip at marker 2q23.3. That one's whispering. Again."

There were emoji reactions, new lines of code, even a moment where Andrew tried to rename their central file from "Attenuation v5" to "The

Ghost Genome." With that, Theo immediately changed it back, replying, "Hard pass. I'm already half-haunted by this dataset."

Some nights, Sonia passes behind Andrew in his home office and gives a wave to the camera. Once, she lingers just long enough to glance at the code on his screen. "You've been at this since five," she murmurs with a motherly tone. "Did you eat?"

Andrew half-smiles and grunts but doesn't answer. Later, when she returns with a sandwich, she hesitates at the door. "You look like you're unraveling something important," she says, while stepping in and setting the plate beside his keyboard. "Just don't unravel with it."

It's the kind of moment that sticks. One that doesn't disrupt the work, and yet gently reminds him there's still a life surrounding it. Sonia catches a glimpse of Andrew's screen where Meera waves an excited greeting through the camera. Sonia offers a warm hello before leaving the room.

The exchange lasts under a minute, but it's enough to leave a silence afterward. A reminder that what they're working on has a weight that tugs beyond spreadsheets and scans. That every theory they test touches real families and real futures.

The cost of their discovery is measured in more than hours. It isn't about disease. It isn't even about damage.

The momentum they've built through data and late-night messages begins to shift into something more urgent. The pieces aren't just aligning. They're starting to implicate systems, rituals, and assumptions far older than science itself.

"There's no shared mutation," Theo says, frustrated. "But the output looks... softened. As if something expected was skipped."

"Every model we've ever built assumes the genome transmits intact," Andrew says, eyes red from hours at the screen. "That deviations are mutations or deletions. But what if something fundamental is just... thinning?"

Theo stops mid-keystroke. "Thinning? Like the ink fading on a copy machine?"

Andrew nodded. "Exactly. The blueprint's still there—sort of—but parts of it are smudged."

Meera taps her pen on the desk. "Which would make sense if we're talking about environmental scaffolding. Not just DNA, but the context around DNA. The microbial network. The ecological memory."

"If that scaffolding starts to fail," Andrew says, "maybe the expression doesn't disappear. It just withers."

Theo responds, half amused. "Okay, but before we start writing science fiction, how are you defining 'thinning'? Because to me, that sounds like code for 'we haven't found the actual variable yet.'"

"It might be," Andrew concedes. "But we've stripped out every obvious factor. The anomalies don't behave like exposure damage or inheritance. They behave like something essential isn't fully arriving."

"Like a delivery missing part of the package," Meera adds.

"Exactly," Andrew says. "The genome shows up. But maybe not the whole system that tells it what to do."

Theo lets out a slow breath. "Okay. Weird. But I'll keep going."

Meera nods slowly, camera flickering from Hyderabad's evening power grid. "Inheritance isn't only about what's passed on," she says. "It's about the environment that supports what's passed. The scaffolding. And scaffolds collapse quietly."

Theo continues while scribbling something on a whiteboard behind him. "You're talking about a signal that fades with each generation. Not just loss. Dampening."

At that moment, Sonia stepped into Andrew's office with a cup of tea in each hand. She glanced at the screen, where the modeling curves and spikes were still visible.

"That looks like my math students on the last week of the semester," she said, setting a mug beside Andrew. "Eager, then drifting. By Friday, they're ghosts."

Theo raised an eyebrow on the video call. "That might be the best summary we've had all day."

Sonia tilted her head, serious now. "You're saying this curve represents inheritance failing, right?"

"Failing softly," Meera replied. "It's erosion more than any kind of rupture."

Sonia nodded. "That reminds me of the way some kids lose language. Not in a dramatic way, just in a slow pullback. A few missed words. Less complexity in their sentences. You don't always see the loss. You feel it."

Andrew looked at her. "Like the genome is doing the same."

Sonia sipped her tea. "So maybe this isn't about what's broken. Maybe it's about what's no longer reinforced. In teaching, if we stop repeating the lesson, kids forget. Why should biology be any different?"

Meera smiled. "I've been thinking about that too. Maybe we're watching what happens when nature stops repeating the right lessons."

They all paused, letting the comparison settle.

"So, we track the shape," Meera continues. "Follow where the drop gets steepest. If the attenuation isn't random, maybe it's a fingerprint. Maybe it's telling us where the signal first starts to break."

Meera's pen freezes midair, her mind suddenly catching on an old memory. When she returns to the present, she sets the pen down and exhales, the room around her silent but for the hum of the monitor. For a moment, she doesn't speak. The image of sterile soil and silent genes lingers, too vivid to ignore.

Andrew notices. "Everything okay?"

Meera nods slowly, then begins to speak. First as a scientist, then as someone piecing together fragments of memory and meaning. She walks them through the Warangal case, step by step. Her voice wavers only once, when she recounts the gel strip that never lit.

It was her third year back in India, after returning from Toronto. She had been investigating a small cluster of pediatric developmental delays in a village outside Warangal. Three children, all born within the same year, presented with eerily similar symptoms. Low muscle tone, delayed speech, and shallow EEG rhythms. There were no common genetic markers, and prenatal care across the families had been consistent. At the time, Meera suspected nutritional deficits or possibly mild perinatal hypoxia, but her conclusions never fully settled.

She had a lingering suspicion, something instinctual and not statistical. During field visits, she'd noticed how local children in one part of the village, those closest to the new cement-lined gravesites, often seemed slower to reach physical milestones than their peers. Parents chalked it up to temperament or family quirks, but Meera couldn't ignore the clustering. Curious whether something in the local environment could be influencing early development, she reached out to a microbiologist at Osmania University. Together, they sampled soil from family compounds and adjacent farmland. What they found startled them. Nearly sterile microbial activity in the soil surrounding the cement-lined burial sites, versus thriving, diverse colonies in nearby plots where traditional, biodegradable burial mats were still used.

The results pushed them further. Partnering with a university lab, they designed a controlled experiment using murine models bred for neurodevelopmental sensitivity. To avoid any ethical ambiguity, they simulated environmental exposure through a sealed chamber system, where the air was enriched with microbial aerosols derived from the contrasting soil samples. One from the sterile burial zone and one from the microbially rich traditional plot. The mice were monitored throughout development, and their offspring were assessed postnatally.

What emerged was subtle but unmistakable. Pups exposed in utero to the aerosolized microbiota from the sterile soil displayed suppressed methylation at specific genomic sites associated with early synaptic development. There were no mutations, no chromosomal breaks. Just silence. Reduced expression. Like instructions half-delivered.

She remembered the moment the data came in. The gel strip didn't light up where it should have. "That's not noise," the technician had said. "That's something we forgot to measure."

Remembering this moment, Meera returns her gaze to Andrew and Theo. She looks up, her voice quieter than before. "I've seen this before. In Warangal. Years ago."

Andrew blinked. "What did you see?"

"Suppressed gene expression. Methylation failures. No apparent failure with DNA transmission, just parts that refused to speak. And the only apparent difference was the microbial profile of the soil around where those children were born."

Theo leaned closer to his screen. "You ran a soil-exposure study?"

Meera nodded. "We thought it was just academic. But now... Now I think it was a fragment of this."

Andrew exhaled. "So, it's not just theory. This has been touched on before. You just didn't recognize what it was."

Theo raised his mug. "Alright, Dr. Rao. You're officially terrifying. Let's keep digging."

Andrew chuckled, catching the double meaning. "You do realize that's the most literal metaphor we've used all day."

Meera smiled, dryly. "Given the topic, I'll allow it."

Theo lets out a slow breath. "Okay. I'll keep going. Just don't make me believe in ghost genes. Not yet. If this turns out to be the next paradigm shift, I'm claiming the title Chief Skeptic Emeritus. I'll even buy a mug to match."

He spins his chair slightly, adding under his breath, "Still not putting glitter on a genome though."

They begin calling it the "Attenuation Curve." A name born from necessity, chosen because no other phrase fits the shape they keep seeing. The moment they name it, something shifts. It stops being an abstraction and becomes a reference point, a shared language. The term begins to appear in their Slack threads, scribbled across Theo's whiteboard, and muttered under Andrew's breath during quiet moments. Meera, who once hesitated to assign a name to something so spectral, finds herself sketching its arc absentmindedly beside her field notes.

Theo still insists the name is a placeholder as they don't fully agree on what it represents yet. Andrew sees it as a shape waiting for context, and Meera calls it a symptom of something older than data. Somehow, naming it changes how they interact with it. The curve gains gravity. It invites questions, demands boundaries, and begins to tether their disparate threads into something unified. For the first time, they aren't just tracking patterns. They're listening to a signal they've acknowledged exists.

The three of them pause under the silence of that acknowledgement. It's reverent. A moment suspended between data points and the first outline of belief.

Each night, they continue to gather their fragments: EEGs, case studies, soil readings, microbial decay rates, and pediatric regression timelines. And each night, someone falters. Once, it's Meera who stares too long at a clustering graph and mutters, "Maybe we're just seeing what we want to see." Another time, Andrew closes his laptop mid-call, rubbing his temples. "What if this is just noise that we've dressed up as signal?"

Even Theo, usually braced in cynicism, goes quiet one evening after running a batch analysis that comes up empty. "I keep expecting a keystone," he says. "Something that makes it all click, but what if it doesn't exist?"

Sometimes, they sit with their doubt.

Inevitably, someone always comes back with a new angle the following morning. A revised overlay. A cleaner filter. It isn't certainty that drives them. It's the shape of the unknown and the sense that, even through fatigue and doubt, something in the pattern is whispering back. None of it should hold together. Yet, through the patterns, it does.

It's a hypothesis rather than proof. One that crosses disciplines and begins to tether them together.

They make no claims. They hold off publishing anything. It feels like it's too early still.

What emerges is more than a dataset. What emerges is a question pulsing beneath everything. What are we failing to inherit? Genetically? Ecologically? Biologically?

If the scaffolding of inheritance is crumbling, how much longer before the blueprint itself no longer makes sense?

Somewhere in northern Finland, a peat-rich graveyard hums with microbial life, nourishing birch trees whose roots have outlived the memory of the buried. In Warangal, a school nurse still wonders why the new children seem quieter than the last. And in Austin, a girl named Junie builds her galaxy out of glitter and string, unaware that her laughter carries the faint echo of everything still fighting to be passed on.

CHAPTER 10
FEEDBACK LOOP

The tipping point arrives after a long silence and an even longer debate.

For Andrew, it begins in an early call with Meera, and Theo still riding the quiet hum of their latest discovery. Theo had just flagged another region in the model showing a near-perfect attenuation slope.

"If we keep this to ourselves much longer," Andrew says, "we're doing more than protecting the theory. We're stalling it."

Meera nods, though her eyes are tired. "We need more data. From outside our loop. From places with different burial norms, different environments. But not a paper. Not yet."

Theo leans back in his chair. "So, we whisper. Not shout. A few forums. Trusted channels. Lead with the data."

Andrew opens a new document. "If someone's going to challenge us, they should be aiming at the model, not the messengers."

Meera taps the table. "Then that's how we do it. Quiet hands. Careful eyes. And just enough signal."

The next day, Theo posts in a private genomics forum: a compressed archive of anonymized case overlays, methylation anomalies, soil correlation graphs, and a note that reads simply, "Open patterns. Interpret responsibly."

Meera shares it with a systems biologist she knows from a global health conference in Nairobi. Andrew forwards it to a pediatric epidemiologist in Toronto, adding only, "You asked for unexplained attenuation patterns? These are ours."

They intentionally withhold broadcasting it like a conclusion. They're opening a question.

The release is controlled to make sure it doesn't go viral. Quiet hands pass the model into underground Slack channels, research backdoors, and fieldworker group chats. The authors aren't named. Just the signal. Just the curve.

In one of those channels, two researchers begin quietly arguing in threaded replies. They debate whether the slope could be an artifact of sample compression. The conversation pulls in others. Someone else posts a counter-model. Yet another overlays environmental metrics that weren't part of the original drop. The discussion grows and maintains the thread without splintering. It deepens without drawing attention to itself or creating a headline. What begins as cautious curiosity becomes a breadcrumb trail of iterative testing.

In a Slack channel for mid-career genomic epidemiologists, a researcher pauses while eating cold noodles at her desk, blinking at the curve Theo posted anonymously. She scrolls back several times. "That can't be noise," she mutters, dragging the window onto her second monitor.

In a secure research backdoor built for peer review exchanges, a junior analyst in Helsinki clicks the archive out of habit and sits forward in his chair as the model loads. He calls his supervisor over with a tone that carries both caution and curiosity. "You might want to see this. I think someone's showing us something we're not supposed to understand yet."

In a WhatsApp group of fieldworkers coordinating maternal health surveys in rural Uganda, a data collector studying fungal colonization in postpartum clinics taps the image open under poor signal and squints. "Wait, this shape," she says aloud, alone in a supply hut. "This looks like the soil maps we thought were broken."

Then the first real response arrived as a direct message from the Netherlands, instead of a comment on the thread, the first true reaction.

It's early morning in Austin when Andrew finds it flagged in his inbox under a science digest subscription he usually ignores. The subject line is understated as it reads, "RE: Pediatric attenuation markers and burial ecology."

The sender catches his eye: Dr. Lotte van Dalen, a bioarchaeologist and population health researcher with the Rijksinstituut voor Volksgezondheid in Utrecht.

She read the preliminary data in the shared model, which was posted anonymously through a collaborative genomic sandbox to which Andrew occasionally contributes. Lotte references their term "attenuation curve" with cautious praise, then offers something bold: twenty-seven years of cross-generational child health data, compiled from her institute's longitudinal mortality archives and municipal land-use records. The link to burial lease cycles emerged only in the last five years, when Lotte began investigating ecological turnover in urban cemeteries as part of a separate population health study. Her data wasn't gathered for this theory, but it fits the shape too well to ignore.

Within a week, they have her on a call. Lotte, pragmatic and precise, immediately questions one part of their model.

"Your interpolation method," she notes. "It assumes a constant rate of ecological decay, as if everything breaks down at the same pace once it's in the ground. But that slope isn't always linear. In regions where burial leases expire at different times, the soil isn't resting between uses. Some plots are reopened while others are still in mid-cycle. That overlap can distort the curve and change how genetic residue reenters the system."

Theo blinks. "You're saying the curve flexes?"

"I'm saying it might. Not everywhere, but in districts where land-use policy changes mid-decade. We have cases like that. I'll send them."

She then explains how Dutch cemeteries recycle grave plots every twenty to thirty years due to limited land.

Theo exhales, half smiling. "So, we've been chasing echoes, and you've been living in the reverberation."

Lotte nods. "If your model is about forgetting, our system is about remembering differently, through reuse."

Meera taps her screen. "Do you have full cohort data?"

"Yes. Child health, burial turnover dates, soil comp analysis, and even fungal loads. We started tracking microfauna in reused plots a few years ago because of urban greening policies. Turns out we already had half your experiment."

Andrew blinks. "Did you know what you were sitting on?"

"Not until your model showed up," Lotte admits. "Once I saw the slope, I couldn't unsee it. I showed it to a colleague. He stared at it for a while and said, 'Looks like we've been composting memory all along.'"

Meera visibly lights up. "So, the body returns fully?"

"Microbially, yes. And legally, unless a family pays to renew the plot, the remains are relocated and the space reused."

Theo raises an eyebrow. "You're saying you've accidentally built the most efficient genetic feedback loop in Europe."

Lotte doesn't smile, but her tone is sincere. "I'm saying your attenuation model might already be reversed here, and I have the pediatric trendlines to test it."

Within two weeks, datasets are moving across three continents.

Late one night, Andrew pauses while reviewing an incoming file from Kerala and mutters, "This is happening faster than we thought possible."

Meera, sipping tea beside him on Zoom, replies, "That's because the signal is speaking to questions they were already asking. We didn't create the need. We just gave it shape."

The second message comes from a university consortium in Japan led by Professor Kaoru Watanabe. His team has been documenting a revival of shizensō—natural forest burials—in the mountainous Gifu Prefecture. Alongside burial records, they've gathered detailed environmental metrics and child health outcomes from nearby villages, originally to explore eco-cultural resilience after depopulation. Their data had sat in isolation, valuable but self-contained, never compared to genomic trends or cross-referenced with global soil assays. Until now, no one had thought to connect patterns of burial renewal with shifts in inherited expression.

Theo scrolls through the attached dataset, his brow furrowing as he scans the headers. "Look at this," he says. "They tracked soil carbon turnover, but they never modeled genetic flux. The samples are clean and deep enough to correlate, if we reprocess them."

Meera nods. "It's the same story everywhere. Environmental scientists track health outcomes. Cultural anthropologists map burial practices. Geneticists focus on expression patterns. Everyone's looking at the same field through their own lens."

Andrew continues the thought. "And no one's asking what happens when those lenses overlap."

The room is quiet for a moment. The idea lands with weight, simple and almost obvious in retrospect. None of the individual studies was wrong; they were just incomplete.

The focus turns back to Kaoru, sitting in front of a simple pine bookcase framed by his camera lens. "When I saw your model, I didn't know whether to feel relieved or unnerved. I thought we were studying cultural revival. Except the curves matched ours more than they should have."

Theo blinks. "Matched how?"

Kaoru pulls up a screen share. "Lichen distribution across burial zones with shizensō rituals. Now look…" he says while overlaying a second chart. "Pediatric neurodevelopmental indices from the same villages. The slope is consistent, even if imperfect."

Meera's eyes light up. "You're saying these are linked?"

"I'm saying," Kaoru replies, "the forest isn't thriving alone. The children are too."

"Were you looking for this?" Andrew asks.

Kaoru shakes his head. "We thought we were measuring cultural resilience. But now, I wonder if we've been documenting an ecological echo. Something the landscape indirectly propagates."

Theo laughs softly. "That's either poetry or the beginning of a new field."

"Both," Kaoru says. "I think it's time we find out which."

Before the month comes to a close, a third message is received from a collaborative lab at the Federal University in São Paulo, led by Dr. Camila Rocha. Her group recently concluded a municipal study on fungal biodiversity around aging cemeteries and informal graveyards. They weren't looking for pediatric trends; however, when Rocha overlaid their environmental samples with public health data, they saw unexpected regional gradients in child development markers.

On a group call, Camila appears with a background of lab freezers and glass-topped petri dishes.

"We've been tracking fungal colonies around São Paulo cemeteries for thirteen years," she says while adjusting her headset. "At first, it was about decay. How humidity and burial style impact surface biodiversity. Then we noticed something odd."

"Odd how?" Theo asks.

Camila clicks through to a slide showing color-coded blocks across a city grid. "Here," she offers. "Fungal richness by cemetery. And now this..." She changes the slide and uses her mouse to point to her scatter plot next to the city grid. "Childhood developmental indices from the nearest public health clinics."

Andrew points. "Those slopes... They match."

Camila nods. "Almost eerily. We saw it first in Vila Formosa, then again in Campo Grande. More biodiversity, better pediatric markers. Less biodiversity. Lower language development. Poorer balance scores."

Meera raises a hand. "Could it be a proxy for pollution? Socioeconomics?"

"We accounted for that. We ran the models ten times over," Camila replies. "It's not a perfect fit, but your attenuation curve gave us a lens we never thought to use."

She pauses, then adds, almost reluctantly. "Something's mediating early childhood brain plasticity. We don't know if it was microbial, chemical, or ancestral. Somehow, your attenuation curve gave us a way to look."

Theo lets out a breath. "Then we're not just chasing ghosts. We're uncovering something threaded through the environment. Signals that aren't random. Instead, they're carried forward in ways we're only starting to understand."

Camila nods. Her tone is thoughtful. "Or maybe it's not just the environment carrying the signal. Maybe we're responding to it. Tuning ourselves without realizing it."

Word is spreading. Quietly. Intently. Avoiding headlines and journals, they find traction in side comments, forwarded links, and long stares at shared monitors. A data coordinator in Kenya forwards the model to her supervisor with the subject line: "You need to see this. It's weird, but it fits." A graduate student in Norway uploads it into a personal data sandbox and spends the night reverse-engineering the trendlines.

Meanwhile, in Austin, Andrew notices more and more flags in the shared document. There are small edits, silent contributors, and footprints left by readers who haven't introduced themselves but have already begun to run calculations.

The coalition begins to form without ever announcing itself.

Andrew tracks the coalition's growth from his office, adding new contributors to the shared grid between patient calls. The list has grown beyond a handful of curious researchers. It's now a patchwork of voices and disciplines from every continent. Lotte van Dalen's Dutch epidemiology team refines longitudinal markers based on burial lease transitions. Kaoru Watanabe's forest-burial cohort in Japan becomes a testbed for ecological continuity metrics. Camila Rocha's lab in São Paulo sends microbial bloom snapshots weekly. Cape Town's pediatric neurodevelopment lab begins a comparative pilot. A small team in Kerala, India, contributes burial exposure data from matrilineal coastal communities, and an Arctic health researcher in Nunavut sends ice-core samples rich in legacy fungal DNA, hoping to draw parallels from permafrost burials.

"New collaborators," Theo mutters, his voice lagging slightly through the video feed. The glow from his monitor flickers across the glassware behind him. "New formats. I swear, some of these files were photographed in candlelight."

"At least yours are digital," Meera says. "Half of these clinic notes are handwritten in dialects even the translators can't agree on. Some are just fragments—phrases, half-sentences, or regional shorthand."

"It's what happens when you pull from rural clinics," Andrew offers. "They document what they can with what they have."

Theo scrolls through a spreadsheet. "I'm building protocol checklists to normalize the entries, but the time zones are a mess. Gifu's nine hours ahead of London, Meera's twelve hours ahead of me, and half these measurements switch between metric and imperial mid-line."

Meera glances at her second screen, stifling a yawn. "I found one blood pressure log written in centimeters for height, inches for arm length, and a note that says, 'stick too short, guessed.'"

Theo laughs. "That's the new control variable. Stick length."

Even Andrew smiles. "We've built models on less."

The humor thins the fatigue, and for a few seconds, the static of the call is the only sound. The distance between them feels almost manageable.

"Still," Meera adds, her tone softening, "we can standardize the numbers, but not the meaning. Each of these entries belongs to a real person, a real place. If we clean too much, we'll erase the story inside it."

Theo nods toward his camera. "Then we adjust the model to the people, not the other way around."

Andrew's voice carries through the speaker with certainty. "That's the point, isn't it? To listen hard enough that the noise stops being noise."

Alongside Andrew, Sonia quietly monitors the communication, watching threads spool and retract, as questions bloom and fade. One night, something catches her attention as she scrolls through a debate about sampling bias in Ugandan soil reports. A data node tagged with a burial zone she studied during her thesis on historical trauma and environmental health. Her pulse ticks up. She re-reads the accompanying notes. It's more than a coincidence.

Sonia's gaze wanders as she thinks through what it would mean if these patterns were more than biological. What if they carried echoes of psychological grief encoded into ritual space? She brings it to Andrew, a bit hesitant. Somewhere in the blur of datasets and drop-ins, Sonia has fully integrated into the conversation and become a full contributor without ever intending to.

She didn't plan to become an active participant. She came to Andrew's office with a simple question: "If the data's real, who explains it to the families?"

He pauses.

"Because if this is more about inheritance than biology. It's a story. It's culture. It's grief."

From that moment, Sonia begins helping shape the communication approach. She conducts communication risk assessments for all information being shared publicly. Even neutral phrases can spark offense across borders. She helps local teams craft culturally specific briefings. Some are rooted in ancestral respect, while others are based on environmental health framing. They identify testing zones by burial practices and microbial composition, as well as linguistic accessibility, historical trauma, and local belief systems.

She teaches the team to move past the analysis and learn to listen. When Meera shares a case from a tribal region in Ghana where a protest erupted over soil sampling in or around burial sites, it was Sonia who helped frame the response. She didn't translate words; she tempered them by guiding the message toward respect and away from defensiveness, keeping the coalition grounded.

"We're doing more than testing hypotheses. We're asking the world to reconsider what it thinks it knows about death, decay, and continuity."

They're building a master dataset. More than that, it's a translation engine for science, mourning, and finding meaning across cultures.

Each country brings its own data and context. Japan has recently revived forest burial rituals in rural prefectures. Brazil brings data on local urban cemeteries showing spikes in congenital anomalies, and one team has already tracked soil nutrient shifts near decomposed human remains.

As the weeks continue to pass, the coalition's work deepens. Andrew builds a comparative map overlay combining burial methods, microbial richness, and pediatric outcomes, layering each new dataset onto the evolving global grid. Theo labels the matrix "Inheritance Scaffold Index," half joking, but their late-night reviews tell a different story. The trendlines are holding, and they grow harder to dismiss with each pass.

One collaborator, Eduardo, a soil fieldworker from São Paulo, shares a video log tracing the edges of urban cemeteries known for poor drainage and overgrowth. In one clip, he stands beside a partially eroded grave wall, gesturing toward fungal clusters emerging through the brickwork.

"Deeper layers show higher microbial respiration," he explains, "but only where the soil is exposed to air and organic exchange. Under concrete vaults, oxygen levels drop sharply, and microbial activity nearly stops." His samples, marked with location codes and moisture readings, confirm the difference in microbial diversity across burial types.

In Japan, Professor Kaoru Watanabe, a cultural anthropologist turned environmental sociologist, leads a quiet revolution in the Gifu Prefecture. There, small communities begin returning to shizensō, natural burials beneath forest canopies. Kaoru's team runs longitudinal child health surveys alongside moss and lichen growth studies. When Meera asks why the two were linked, Kaoru explains, "We don't separate what grows above and what grows within. When families bury their dead in the forest, the trees inherit them too."

Not every contribution goes smoothly. During one call, a French bioethicist in the coalition expresses unease about the theory's implications. "You're venturing into sacred ground, literally and philosophically," she warns. "You risk unraveling people's sense of what death means." The warning lands as both caution and proof. The discomfort itself means they're asking the right questions.

Theo responds first, his voice unusually measured. "Then we need to treat this as more than a model. If we're right, it's a measure of interdependence within genetics. Disrupt enough relationships in an ecosystem, and even the strongest patterns can unravel."

Sonia follows gently. "It still matters that we asked, even if we're wrong."

That conversation prompts the coalition to pause. To challenge themselves harder. They form a new working subgroup to test for researcher bias, confirmation bias, and confounding variables. Meera drafts a set of blind validation protocols. Theo insists on replication by outside labs. He outlines a triple-blind cohort replication where even the analysts won't know which datasets come from presumed attenuation zones.

A team in Cape Town takes the first replication test. Their results mirror the attenuation curves in two of the four control groups. Even though it's not a perfect alignment, the results are close enough to lend weight. They remain cautious, just the same. A second lab in Vancouver finds no meaningful curve, citing inconsistencies in soil sampling techniques. Rather than dismiss the result, the coalition folds the critique into the next round.

Kaoru raises a cultural warning: "Some zones may not exhibit attenuation because their ritual ecology has never been broken. The soil has never experienced absence."

Eduardo agrees. "Some cities in Brazil have had sealed tombs for less than thirty years. The legacy isn't deep enough. You're looking for a wound that hasn't scarred yet."

The group compiles a catalog of confounds: soil acidity, rainfall patterns, fungal interference, cultural burial exceptions, and industrial zoning. They run simulations with each variable suppressed and again with each amplified. In one version, Sonia has them replace all burial language with the neutral phrasing, "residual nutrient discontinuity," and "post-mortem microbial sequestration," to see if the bias lingers when the metaphor disappears.

It did. The attenuation signal still pulsed.

Still, they aren't ready to accept it without challenge. The implications are too wide and too easily misunderstood. They rotate datasets between national teams and anonymized regional flags, testing for consistency, bias, and edge-case anomalies. Theo color-codes every file with a confidence score, a running audit of how bold each leap in interpretation has become.

By the end of the following month, they've ruled out over sixty potential confounds.

Accounted for in the results, even if they aren't eliminated entirely.

With each audit, the pattern grows clearer.

Nonetheless, clarity brings scrutiny. Fortunately, it's not from outside critics, at least not yet. The scrutiny comes from within.

It begins with a message from a Quebec researcher who initially helped source pediatric EEG baselines. The message is polite, while at the same time, tense. "You're pushing too close to cultural contamination. Be careful. This smells like epigenetic determinism if the wrong person reads it."

Meera reads it slowly, then forwards it to the group with the added line, "We need to talk about framing."

The debate fractures the coalition's usually fluid rhythm. One heated message from a South African contributor accuses another of "scientific colonialism," not for changing any practice but for interpreting Indigenous burial records through a Western frame of reference. The concern isn't about the data itself but about ownership. Who defines meaning, and who speaks for the dead? Another thread spins out as a Brazilian contributor warns of cultural erasure, the fear that context will be lost once numbers replace narrative.

Theo tries to moderate, but his tone sharpens. Kaoru goes silent. The chat stalls.

Then Sonia intervenes. She reframes the argument by anchoring it in shared stakes, not in who speaks loudest, but in who might suffer most if they get it wrong. She invites each critic to rephrase their concern as a guiding question, and slowly, the conversation reopens. Some collaborators argue that avoiding controversy is cowardice. Others warn that if they aren't precise in their language, the work could be co-opted by nationalists, traditionalists, or worse.

Andrew calls an emergency roundtable. Sonia moderates.

"I want us to imagine," she says, "that someone publishes a response before we're ready. They twist our model into something harmful. What would they use? What would they say?"

"They'd say we're ranking cultures by genetic hygiene," Theo replies, "or that we're implying sealed burials create defective children."

Kaoru winced. "This is why we need to be exact in how we frame it," he said. "Burial practices are part of the pattern, yes. But publicly, we should speak about environmental interruption and not ritual. We're exploring how natural cycles degrade when they're sealed off, not how anyone grieves."

Eduardo finally grounds the tension. He recounts a site in Recife where multiple families have resisted cemetery renovation because they believe the new vaults are suffocating tree roots more than any cultural reason.

"They didn't have our data," he admits. "Still, they felt something was wrong. We aren't inventing a new belief. We're rediscovering one that people have already sensed."

The room falls quiet. Sonia nods.

"We're still asking the same thing," she says, "but we need to ask it like the world is listening now."

Just as the coalition begins speaking more carefully, others start to listen.

CHAPTER 11
SCAFFOLDS OF THE EARTH

The first real break in their assumptions came from historical records. There's evidence that resists explanation.

Theo finds it buried in a footnote. He's reviewing an old demographic paper from the University of Edinburgh, a preprint from the early 2000s that modeled childhood mortality in post-famine Ireland. It's late, but he's curious. The impact of the footnote stops him cold.

"Recovery in pediatric vitality observed within two generations of the 1840s famine. DNA fragments from naturally buried remains in western Ireland show shifts in gene frequency and stress-linked methylation patterns, hinting at enhanced developmental stability in the post-famine population."

His eyes stay affixed to the screen for a moment, unblinking. Then he opens a message to Meera and Andrew.

Theo writes one line: "Check pg 112, fn.7. If this is real, we just found our first backward echo."

Even after sending the message, Theo doesn't move. He scrolls back up and re-reads the footnote. He isn't sure if it's the hour or the implication, but his chest tightens. A signal? No. Not possible. Not like this.

Yet he feels the ripple beneath his rationality. The precision of the phrasing needles at his certainty. He's seen enough scientific prose to know when language reaches beyond data. This whisper, wrapped in evidence and waiting to be heard, carries the weight of something undeniable—more origin than guesswork.

He sets down his mug. His hand trembles slightly as he navigates back through the document. He tries to dismiss the thoughts of confirmation bias or late-night pattern recognition, but it sticks.

Because what if this wasn't an anomaly?

He flips through the bibliography and follows the citation trail. One link is dead. Another leads to a scan of a yellowed field report. It's a catalog of soil stratification data, mineral loss, and a side note on femoral density ratios in juvenile remains. Theo points to the screen. There it is: higher-than-expected cortical bone thickness, stronger tooth enamel, no evidence of preservative chemicals. The children were buried quickly, directly, and without ritual.

He opens a new tab and begins pulling nutritional records, infant mortality rates, and burial site topography overlays from the supplementary data. He searches without answers. Something waits in the silence. He can feel it.

By the time Andrew opens the file, Theo has already pulled the original excavation reports. Meera chimes in within the hour.

"The bones were never preserved for pathology. Isotope analysis reveals elevated prenatal nutrition markers and higher bone density, and they were buried in unsealed ground, without stone or sealant."

Andrew scans the summary. "That doesn't make sense. A mass death event typically correlates with worse health, not improved outcomes."

"Unless," Meera says softly, "something about the burial ecology reset the system."

Theo continues reading from the article. "The famine devastated Ireland's population, but by necessity, bodies were returned to the earth in the simplest way imaginable. No vaults. No embalming. Just cloth, soil, and time. In the generations that followed, regions that practiced natural burial showed subtle upticks in developmental resilience among surviving children. Not everywhere, but where the ground was left open, the gains appeared."

"It's a reversal of everything we've been told," Andrew says in mild protest. "Vaults, concrete, and containment were meant to protect the living from the dead. But maybe the danger wasn't the microbes."

Meera nods. "We keep assuming contamination. But what if what's being lost isn't infectious? It's instructive. The microflora, the mineral exchange, the gene fragments completing the cycle."

Andrew glances at the data. "So, what we've been sealing away is information."

"The pattern isn't limited to Europe," Meera continues, already ahead of them. "During the Dust Bowl of the 1930s, which affected the southern Great Plains, including parts of Texas, Oklahoma, and Kansas, entire communities buried their dead directly in the eroded ground. There were no vaults, no preservatives, just soil stripped bare by drought and wind. For many, it was a necessity. Those who stayed had no choice but to return the bodies quickly, before the next storm buried them in dust."

She scrolls through a weathered regional report. "Most families eventually left, heading west toward California, but some returned a decade later when the rains came back. And here's what's strange: in counties that repopulated after the drought, public health records show a quiet rebound. There were higher infant survival rates and fewer congenital complications. It's as if the land, after losing so much, began to recalibrate. Where the soil was allowed to heal naturally, life adapted faster."

Andrew rubs his temple. "So, mass tragedy may have triggered micro-ecological resets."

He pauses, then adds, "Like the genome got a reboot through the soil. As if the ground itself remembered how to rebuild, only when unburdened by our fear of decay."

Theo pulls up a chart. "Every time we trace the data, the same arc appears. Crisis. Collapse. Return to natural burial. Then drift correction. Even if we prove the signal exists, where's the connection? How is this leading to improved outcomes?"

"First, we prove it's real," Meera suggests. "Then we ask what it means."

Everyone takes a moment to consider this. Even the sound of shifting papers stops. For the first time, the enormity of what they're chasing feels tangible, a question that reaches beyond science. Each of them knows that meaning will come with risk and that discovery, once named, can't be undone.

Until now, Sonia has been observing the conversation develop while she and Andrew finish breakfast at their kitchen counter, both staring at Andrew's laptop.

She asks the obvious follow-up question. "If natural burial leads to drift correction, however that happens, what does that say about our rituals? Our need to preserve?"

The group remained quiet in their shared contemplation. These questions tug at the heart of the matter. What's the true cause, and what's the outcome likely to look like?

Andrew breaks the silence, his voice low. "It says what we call dignity might come at a cost we never measured."

With that, the group breaks.

Later that night, Sonia sits with Andrew by the glow of a dim kitchen light. A half-eaten biscuit rests on a napkin between them. The tea has gone tepid. She traces the rim of her cup with slow, rhythmic circles, the ceramic warm beneath her fingertips.

"I remember my grandmother's funeral," she says. "We buried her in a vault lined with pink granite. She would've hated it. She used to say, 'Let the worms do their work. I don't need to be frozen in stone.' But my aunt insisted. She said we owed her something lasting."

The silence that follows feels like it's charged. Sonia's gaze drifts toward the window, but her focus is somewhere deeper.

Andrew tilts his head. "Did anyone fight it?"

Sonia lets out a breath, more sigh than breath. "My mother didn't want to argue. Everyone was grieving. Besides, it felt... respectful. That was the word everyone used."

"Just not the word she would've chosen," Andrew says softly.

"No." Her voice is firmer now, more certain. "She wanted a simple cloth and wildflowers. She made us promise once, in passing. However, no one could bring themselves to do it when it came time. We needed something that felt permanent. We wanted to hold on."

She presses the rim of the cup to her lip but doesn't drink. "I think I knew even then that it wasn't for her. It was for us. To feel like we had done something. Controlled something. That we hadn't lost everything."

She looks out the window. "Maybe it's not the dead who need protection. Maybe it's us."

Two weeks later, Andrew presents a subset of their anonymized data at a small roundtable on ecological inheritance hosted in Oslo. Halfway through the talk, a well-known geneticist from Denmark stands up.

"You're suggesting that unregulated death is a public good," she states flatly. "That's barbarism dressed in biology. That's not science."

Andrew holds her gaze. "I'm saying we might have mistaken sterility for respect. If our preservation methods disrupt inheritance, then we must ask what we're actually preserving."

She turns to the audience. "This is dangerous language. It undermines centuries of ritual."

"And yet," Meera adds from her seat, "so does the data."

Another attendee, an anthropologist from Istanbul, raises a hand. "Maybe the question isn't whether the theory offends tradition. Maybe it's whether we have the courage to update it."

After the session, the Danish geneticist approaches Andrew privately.

"I lost my mother last year," she says quietly. "She was embalmed. Buried in stone. Now you're telling me that might have hurt the Earth she loved."

Andrew softens. "I'm telling you we don't know. We're trying to ask the question no one wanted to ask. Because if there's a chance, even a small one, that we can restore something we've broken... don't you want to know too?"

She doesn't answer. She just walks away quietly.

The more they look, the more the pattern emerges.

In Rwanda, post-genocide burial fields with unembalmed mass graves showed, a decade later, higher than expected rates of neonatal vitality.

In Ukraine, early Soviet-era trench burials during the Holodomor are now part of an ecological restoration project. One researcher noted that the trees planted above those sites have stronger fungal symbiosis than the surrounding areas.

In Chile, post-earthquake communities forced to bury the dead without coffins saw unusual longevity in pediatric populations up to two generations later.

Still, not everyone is convinced.

Sonia sits back from the map, arms folded. She's been quiet for most of the discussion, listening the way she always does when the room starts circling its own brilliance. "It's compelling," she says, "but correlation isn't causation. What if this is just an artifact? Noise we've mistaken for structure?"

Theo glances at her, half-smiling. "Leave it to the non-scientist to ask the one question that keeps us honest. We've controlled for dozens of variables. But sure, we can't rule out unseen confounds."

Meera adds gently, "That's why we test. It's good to be cautious. We can't afford premature conclusions."

Sonia nods. "Then let's keep checking. I just don't want the narrative to outrun the evidence."

Theo begins calling the trend points "the forgiveness zones."

Meera hates the term. "The earth doesn't forgive. It integrates. We need to stop romanticizing the recovery. It was born of horror."

Theo nods. "Point taken. Still, the trendline holds."

Andrew looks at the map. Dozens of red pins dot it now. Places where, through tragedy, burial returned to something raw. Meanwhile, the generations that followed showed strange upticks in resilience.

He traces his finger across the screen.

"Is it possible," he whispers, "that catastrophe corrected something we broke on purpose?"

Sonia, reading behind him, says softly, "Maybe it's not correction. Maybe it's just recalling what was already there."

Andrew glances up. "Recalling?"

"Not memory, exactly," she says. "More like the soil remembering its balance — the way ecosystems fall back into rhythm when we stop interfering."

Still, not all loss nourishes the soil. Some silenced it.

Then Cambodia.

It's Meera who opens the door. She's been corresponding with a team from Phnom Penh University, where a small group of researchers were digitizing burial site data from the Khmer Rouge era. Between 1975 and 1979, nearly two million people, roughly a quarter of Cambodia's population, were executed or starved to death under Pol Pot's regime. Most were buried in mass graves, shallow and hastily dug, in what became known as the Killing Fields.

The research team, led by Dr. Vannary Keo, was not initially studying genetics. Their work focused on preserving testimony and identifying remains. However, over the past decade, Dr. Keo noticed something in the longitudinal health data of children born in surrounding villages.

"We weren't looking for drift," she explains to Meera in a late-night video call. "But our pediatric health curves... They were unusual."

"How?" Andrew asks, leaning into the screen.

"Cognitive markers. Language acquisition. Immunity response. In regions adjacent to the graves, the next generation of children showed slightly elevated developmental resilience. Nothing dramatic. Just a quiet curve, moving upward."

Theo frowns. "Could it be statistical noise? Survivorship bias?"

"We thought so too," Vannary admits. "We controlled for displacement, malnutrition, and even education. It kept showing up. When we mapped soil microbiota in those same regions..."

She flips the camera to her screen. Spore colonies. Microbial bloom rates. Methylation field overlays.

"We found a significant microbial rebound. The graves weren't sealed. There was no preservation. Bodies were returned fully to the earth, and something about that echoed forward."

Silence hung between them.

"You think this is inheritance," she states, not as a question.

"No," Meera interjects before Vannary can reply. "I think it's what makes inheritance possible."

Vannary looks down for a moment. When she looks up again, her voice cracks.

"My uncle was buried in one of those fields. He was seventeen. We never found him, but if this is true, if something good came from that horror, then maybe there's something we can still carry forward."

Andrew nods, blinking away the signs of his emotion.

"That's all we're trying to do," he says. "We're not rewriting the past. We're listening to what it's trying to teach us."

Not all tragedies lead to renewal.

In 2014, as Ebola spread across West Africa, governments and health agencies enforced strict burial protocols to contain the virus. Bodies were sealed in impermeable plastic shrouds, sometimes double-wrapped, and buried deep in specially designated sites, far from community land. Contact was forbidden. In many regions, traditional rites were suspended. Grieving families could not touch or wash the bodies. Many never saw them again.

A research team in Sierra Leone, led by Dr. Aminata Kamara, was studying post-epidemic community health due to this tragedy when she came across the attenuation theory. She reached out.

"We wanted to know if there had been any rebound. Like what you saw in Bulgaria or India," she says to Theo over a choppy connection.

Theo probes, "And?"

Aminata's voice is tight. "There wasn't. If anything, developmental health metrics declined. Not from trauma alone. We accounted for that."

"What changed?" he asked.

"The soil," she offers. "The microbial sampling from the burial fields was sterile. Almost inert. Nothing grew above the plastic-shrouded plots. Not even weeds."

"It had to be," Meera says quietly. "Ebola containment, full isolation — no chance for leakage." She pauses, watching the data scroll. "But the irony is, the same safeguards that protected the living erased the ecology underneath."

Andrew struggles to find his voice and coughs to clear it. "The feed-back loop was broken," he offers, less as a question and more as a statement.

Aminata nods. "We thought we were containing the infection. We did, but in doing so, we may have severed something else."

For a moment, no one speaks. Then Sonia, staring at the map in front of her, whispers, "We were trying to save lives, and in the process, we cut off what connected us to them."

Meera looks up. "We inadvertently cut off the exchange that used to pass quietly back through the soil. The microbes, minerals, and fragments of DNA that once fed the system. We stopped the transfer."

Theo closes his eyes. "We treated the ground like a vault. Locked it. Sealed it. As a result, now it's gone silent."

Andrew taps the edge of the table, thinking aloud. "What if this silence is the cost? More than the absence of bloom, the loss of something still beyond our ability to measure?"

Aminata's voice, when it returns, is softer. "We did what we had to, but science demands we ask the question, 'At what price?'"

They all sit with the weight of it. Not guilt or blame. The slow, sobering recognition that in trying to protect one part of life, they may have amputated another.

The same pattern appeared in early COVID-era burials. In New York City, overwhelmed morgues resorted to mass graves on Hart Island. Many bodies, especially during the spring of 2020, were placed in sealed plastic body bags and buried in bulk. Identification was delayed or lost. Families were not allowed to gather.

In India, footage from Delhi and Mumbai shows overrun crematoriums and hastily dug burial trenches. Health workers wrapped the deceased in multiple layers of synthetic material to prevent viral transmission. Bodies were placed in cement-lined pits, and in some cases, doused with chemicals.

Soil samples from these zones, now quietly studied by environmental labs, show signs of microbial stasis.

Meera says it first: "No bloom."

Theo responds, "Just void."

Sonia sits beside Andrew, scrolling through photos from the Delhi fieldwork. Her voice is soft. "We left nothing for the soil to work with. Our focus was solely on protecting the living."

Andrew looks up. "Which means we need to rethink the whole system. Honoring the dead and protecting the yet-to-be-born as part of the same continuum."

The coalition meets in a private virtual conference room two nights later. Nearly a dozen small windows light the screen: Tokyo, Utrecht,

Pune, São Paulo, Austin, Kigali, Helsinki. Time zones be damned, they're all awake.

Theo opens with a scan of a slide. No labels. Just a single sine wave overlaid with red points. The attenuation curve.

"We've seen enough to ask the next question," he says. "Wherever burial is sealed, the soil falls quiet. Wherever the dead return fully, something echoes forward. It's more than a theory. This is a pattern."

Camila Rocha leans in. "It's not universal. Not yet. We've got contradictions. Outliers. No consistent measurement standard."

Andrew nods. "That's why we need more data. Starting with the past. We need to test the signal across time, cultures, and continents."

Meera pulls up a shared document titled, *Retrospective Global Soil Health Study.*

"This is our proposal," she says. "We draw on historical burial records, digitized grave maps, and old agricultural plots that intersect with known unsealed and sealed interment sites. We sample the soil. We track the microbial biodiversity. We overlay pediatric health metrics."

Lotte van Dalen is already nodding while saying, "The Netherlands has eighty years of cemetery lease data. I can provide microbial samples from recycled plots dating back to the 1950s."

Kaoru adds, "We can integrate shizensō regions in Gifu Prefecture. They've had forest burials uninterrupted for three generations. Child health surveys are available."

"Sor—, São Paulo, —ld you repeat that?" The call lagged, fragmenting Camila's voice.

"We're seeing early-stage data that doesn't match the pattern," she says again. "A site in the Amazon where bodies were returned to the earth, but the fungal load never took. No signal. No bloom."

Theo frowns. "Maybe climate extremes suppressed the ecology?"

"Maybe," Kaoru offers, "it's not just how we bury. It's how we live before we die."

Camila raises a finger. "We'll need strict controls. Variables like socioeconomic status, rainfall, industrial zoning, and soil pH all need to be tracked. We must ensure full anonymization. If raw data circulates without safeguards, someone will find a way to misuse it."

Sonia, who's been quiet until now, speaks up. "We'll need narrative alignment. If this becomes about who buries better, we've already failed."

Andrew glances around the screen. "We agree this doesn't get published yet. Not until we've tested the hypothesis through neutral labs. Multiple samples. Verified overlap."

Kaoru nods. "Science first. Story later."

Meera adds, "We should prioritize zones with existing pediatric cohort studies. We can anonymize the regions and assign numerical IDs. No names. No rituals. Just soil and signal."

Theo's already typing. "We'll need a centralized index. I'll draft the schema. Markers include microbial load, mycorrhizal diversity, and dominant bacterial species. Tie them to burial type, time since decomposition, and longitudinal child health markers."

Aminata Kamara from Sierra Leone lifts her voice. "I'll oversee post-epidemic zones, but I want trauma-screening protocols in place. No study goes forward unless families in those regions are consulted."

Sonia looks up. "The language we use shapes the work. This study reaches beyond biology and engages with the persistence of life through soil and cycle."

Kaoru smiles gently. "Then let's treat memory with the care we give a genome. With dignity."

Andrew closes the meeting with a single question.

"If this study confirms what we suspect, if the scaffolding of inheritance is ecological as much as it is genetic, then what are we willing to do with that truth?"

He doesn't expect an answer. Not yet. Somehow, the silence on screen feels louder than any vow. Lotte shifts slightly in her seat, eyes darting away from the camera. Kaoru stares forward, unblinking, as if translating the weight of the question into something she can carry. Theo rubs the bridge of his nose, then closes his laptop slowly but doesn't disconnect. Sonia, caught mid-thought, looks like she's about to speak but doesn't. Her gaze lingers on the screen a moment longer before the window minimizes into darkness.

Still, no one logs off.

That night, long after Sonia had gone to bed, Andrew opened his private notes.

He stares at the blinking cursor, unsure where to begin. The screen glows in the silence, throwing pale light across the kitchen counter.

"If the hypothesis holds," he types, "then our species has been severing something it never knew it needed. All in the name of cleanliness. Honor. Memory."

He pauses.

"What if the loss we associate with decay is actually a transfer of function—nutrient cycles resetting, microbial networks rebalancing? Our burial practices may have disrupted the very feedback loops that sustain ecological and developmental health."

He sits back and rereads the lines. They carry the weight of something significant. A beginning.

CHAPTER 12
BURIED SIGNALS

The confrontation happens in the small, wood-paneled conference room near the administrative wing of Dell Children's. Andrew arrives first, adjusting the collar of his white coat and scanning the empty chairs. He carries a folder thick with notes, highlighted EEG charts, and anonymized patient logs. Theo arrives moments later, tieless and tense, with a laptop tucked under one arm and an energy drink in the other. He offers Andrew a glance that says, *Let them come.*

Dr. Miriam Kline, Head of Pediatric Neurology, enters with a practiced smile. She's joined by Harold Brenner, the hospital's Director of Research Oversight. They sit across from Andrew and Theo, hands folded, expressions neutral.

"Dr. Turbin. Dr. Manning," Miriam begins. "Thank you for joining us. We've been reviewing departmental expenditures and noticed some unusual upticks in sequencing requests, research software licenses, and fieldwork reimbursements."

Andrew meets her gaze. "All authorized within our departmental scope. The fieldwork costs were shared with my colleagues overseas. We're collaborating on a multi-institutional study."

Harold clears his throat. "Which brings us to the concern. This research crosses into sensitive territory. Cultural, religious, and even ethical. The language used in your draft proposals is troubling to some of our advisory reviewers."

"You're referring to the hypothesis about ecological inheritance and burial ecology?" Theo asks.

"We're referring to the implication that our current burial practices may be biologically disruptive," Harold replies. "That's not a conclusion this institution is prepared to endorse."

Andrew opens his folder. "We're not drawing conclusions. We're identifying a pattern. EEG anomalies, attenuation curves, and transgenerational expression irregularities. They all point toward a systemic disruption. We believe soil ecology plays a role."

Miriam interrupts. "We understand the science, Dr. Turbin. What we're concerned about is the messaging. This hospital is not positioned to withstand the kind of scrutiny that comes from challenging funerary traditions."

"Scrutiny from who?" Theo asks. "Religious groups? Lobbyists? Cemetery boards? This is data. We're not introducing doctrine."

Harold raises a hand. "Dr. Manning, this isn't just about scientific accuracy. It's about institutional risk. You're both respected physicians. The optics of your theory linking childhood neurodevelopment to burial practices are incendiary."

Andrew draws in a slow breath. "We're not making a political statement. We're asking a biological question. The signal in the data demands investigation."

Miriam looks down at a printed copy of their abstract. "Your phrase here, 'sealed burial halts microbial reintegration,' was flagged by multiple reviewers."

"Because it's accurate," Theo replies. "The soil depends on that reintegration to maintain its biological network."

"The perception matters," Harold says. "Public trust is fragile. This institution serves families from many faiths. If we appear to challenge their mourning rituals, we may lose more than grant funding. We could lose our community."

"What happens when those families start asking why their children are sick," Andrew interrupts, "and we had an answer and didn't look into it? I'm happy to avoid the headlines while we continue to study the mechanism. Quietly. Rigorously. Respectfully."

Miriam exhales. "We're not asking you to abandon the work, but we are instituting oversight. Effective immediately, our Ethics Committee must approve any research activities related to this theory. No travel, no publications, no external collaboration without prior clearance."

"So, we're muzzled," Theo mutters.

Harold frowns. "You're guided. We're trying to protect you and the hospital."

Andrew lifts a page from his folder and lays it gently on the table. It's a scatterplot showing EEG attenuation curves overlaid with methylation patterns from a dozen pediatric cases. Each one shows drift.

"We're past theoretical," he says. "This is already happening. Something is missing in the biology of our patients. We must consider that our current medical, ecological, or cultural systems may be contributing to that loss."

Miriam studies the chart in silence, her expression unreadable.

"You're asking us to support a theory that rewrites the relationship between death and biology," she says quietly.

"No," Andrew replies. "We're asking you to help us listen to the Earth. Because it's trying to tell us something."

Harold shifts in his seat. "If you continue, understand that you carry this risk personally. The institution will not shield you from reputational fallout."

Theo offers plainly, arms crossed. "Then we'll carry it, but don't pretend caution is the same as safety. Ignoring a signal doesn't make it go away."

Miriam nods slowly. "Then tread carefully. Science at this level is a double-edged sword. You may discover something true, but not all truth is welcome."

Andrew closes the folder. "We're seeking truth more than we're looking for approval. What matters here is what's real."

Harold offers a final warning glance. "Then be sure you're ready to live with what you find."

They exit the room into a sterile hallway, white walls and linoleum stretching endlessly in both directions. Theo exhales sharply.

"Well," he mutters, "that could've gone worse."

Andrew raises an eyebrow. "Really?"

"Okay, it went exactly as badly as I expected. At least we're not fired."

Andrew laughs under his breath, stopping outside the pediatric ICU. Through the glass, machines breathe for their patients.

"They don't see it yet," he says.

"They will," Theo answers. "The evidence will catch up."

Andrew glances once more toward the ward before turning back toward the lab, the hum of ventilators fading behind him.

That night, Meera joins them on a secure call from her office. The low hum of an overhead fan buzzes faintly through her speaker, and behind her, the tall shelves of medical records cast long shadows in the soft lamp glow.

Her expression sharpens when Andrew relays the news.

"You didn't tell them?!" she asks sharply.

"We didn't think it would move this fast," Andrew replies, his voice taut with frustration. "They saw the expense trail and jumped."

Theo chimes in. "Apparently, we're going to start a religious revolution if we sequence more soil."

Meera folds her arms. "This theory challenges deeply held beliefs. You can't afford to be opaque. I brought my department chair into the loop months ago. They didn't like it, but they respected the transparency."

"What did you tell them?" Andrew asks.

Meera sits back in her chair, recalling. "I scheduled a quiet meeting with the hospital's ethics board and my department chair. I presented the data gently, not the full theory, not at first. I focused on the anomalies. Birth defect patterns, the ecological drift, and the microbial diversity gaps. I framed it as a question of systems."

Theo raises an eyebrow. "And they didn't throw you out of the room?"

"They asked hard questions," Meera says. "They wanted to know what we were implying. Whether we were suggesting that cultural burial rites were harming future generations. Whether the research could be misused by nationalist agendas. Whether grieving families might be blamed for the choices they made."

Andrew nods grimly. "Same here. They're worried about optics. About upsetting religious communities. About the hospital looking like it's dictating how people should honor their dead."

"Exactly," Meera says. "So, I told them we weren't seeking to blame anyone or assign fault. We're trying to understand if an ecological mechanism exists that no one has noticed. If the soil plays a role in how life reseeds itself, then we owe it to science and to our patients to investigate."

"And they bought that?" Andrew asks with a bit of shock in his voice.

"They didn't embrace it," Meera says. "But they allowed it. I'm under soft oversight now, including quarterly summaries to the ethics panel, and pre-approval for any published language. They didn't object to the data, only to how I framed it."

Andrew frowns. "Framed it how?"

"I used to write the way we talked when the work was still exploratory. Sacred disruption, memory in the soil, echoes of the dead. They said it blurred the line between observation and belief. Now I have to translate everything into neutral terms: 'attenuation patterns in microbial biodiversity linked to interment infrastructure.'"

Theo groans. "That sounds like a grant proposal written by AI."

"Nevertheless, it passed," Meera says, half smiling. "When the phrasing is clinical, they stop asking questions. The language protects the work."

Andrew exhales. "So, we walk a tightrope. Say enough to keep moving forward, but not enough to draw fire."

"Exactly," Meera replies. "If we describe it as an emerging pattern needing validation, they nod. If we describe it as evidence of something deeper, they panic."

Theo taps his pencil. "Then we standardize the language into a shared glossary, so we're consistent."

Meera turns her camera toward a spiral notebook filled with two columns. "Already started. Left side: how we actually talk. Right side: the versions that get past committees."

"So, we translate ourselves to stay viable," Theo summarizes.

Meera nods. "That's the cost of keeping the research alive."

Andrew watches the screen for a long moment. "Then let's be precise. If clarity buys us time, we use it. The work matters more than the wording."

No one disagrees.

Meera continues, "We need to be clear-eyed. If this theory gains traction, it will upset people. It challenges how they define legacy and invites them to see it through a new lens."

Theo nods. "If we don't control the story, someone else will, and they won't be careful."

Andrew folds his hands. "So, we stay cautious. Transparent. Collaborative. We build the U.S/scaffolding and let the weight of evidence do the work without drawing undo attention to it."

Meera agrees. "We keep each other honest. If any of us pushes the boundary too far, the others pull back. We are each other's oversight."

Theo lifts his mug in a half-salute. "To being the world's most cautious revolutionaries."

Meera raises an eyebrow. "Let's just be the most precise. The revolution will come later."

They share a quiet moment on screen. Three researchers in their own corner of the world, one fragile theory wrapped in data, doubt, and dangerous possibility.

Theo breaks the silence first. "Okay. If we're moving forward, we need the next site. We need a long-term burial ground with minimal interference. Somewhere, we can measure decades of decay and microbial inheritance."

"Preferably with variation in burial methods," Meera adds. "Embalmed versus unembalmed. Vaulted versus non-vaulted."

Andrew nods, tapping a pen against his desk. "We also need geographic diversity. Something in a temperate climate, ideally. Not too dry, not too acidic."

"India won't work," Meera says. "Cremation is the dominant practice, and even where burial occurs, the records are spotty. Plus, monsoon variability disrupts soil continuity."

"The U.S. has decent data," Theo offers. "But the modern cemeteries here use too many vaults. Too much sealing. We'd be studying concrete rather than decomposition."

"Eastern Europe?" Andrew suggests. "Post-Soviet cemeteries sometimes lacked preservation materials."

"Unfortunately, the recordkeeping is inconsistent," Meera counters. "And politically sensitive right now. We'd be under scrutiny from the start."

Theo scratches his head. "What about South America? Argentina? Rural cemeteries from the early twentieth century might have natural conditions."

"We'd run into biological noise," Andrew says. "High fungal activity. Also, legal permissions would take years."

They sit in silence for a moment, each scrolling through mental maps, archives, and microbiomes.

Then Andrew's eyes flicker. "Normandy. The D-Day cemeteries."

Meera blinks. "That's sacred ground."

"Exactly," he says. "Thousands of bodies. Minimal embalming. Biodegradable caskets. Natural decay in post-war soil."

Theo pauses before continuing. "The records should be meticulous. Burial plots are aligned with unit data. Locations, dates of death, even cause in some cases."

Meera tilts her head. "That might actually work. You get the decay profile of soldiers from multiple nations, buried in roughly the same window. Different genetics. Different cultural funeral norms with consistent site conditions."

"We'd have to get permissions from the French Ministry of Culture, the U.S. Department of Veterans Affairs, and likely German consulates as well," Andrew says. "Plus, local authorities and custodians of the cemeteries themselves."

"We'll need to include the religious representatives," Meera adds. "Don't forget them."

"It'll be a bureaucratic nightmare," Theo concedes. "But the soil... The soil might speak more clearly than any we've touched."

They move forward with determination, undeterred by the bureaucratic gauntlet ahead.

Over the next six months, the trio becomes both scientists and diplomats. They draft formal petitions in triplicate, labor through Zoom calls with translators, and submit documentation into black-hole portals operated by foreign bureaucracies.

Meera scrolls through the latest reply from Paris and exhales. "The Ministry wants us to justify the scientific value again without suggesting we dishonor the fallen." She reads aloud, "The tone is clinical, but insufficiently reverent."

Theo leans over her shoulder. "So, we're supposed to sound reverent while discussing microbial decay?"

"Apparently," she says. "They'll only sign off if we make the purpose sound like an act of preservation."

Andrew rubs his forehead. "Then let's give them that. 'Preservation of legacy through biological stewardship.' It's true enough, and it might keep them happy."

Three days later, France grants tentative approval.

Across the table, Andrew opens the U.S. response. "Veterans Affairs wants to know if we're disturbing any headstones, flower beds, or nearby graves. They want photographs of the equipment."

Theo slides a soccer ball across the floor toward him. "For scale," he grins.

Andrew takes the photo, then adds a note: non-invasive sampling; surface depth limited to thirty centimeters.

Meera looks up. "Should I send a thank-you if they approve?"

"Handwritten," Andrew says. "They'll appreciate the gesture."

Germany's reply arrives next. Meera reads it aloud: "They're cooperative, but they want full chain-of-custody documentation for where every sample goes, how it's stored, and how DNA fragments are treated."

Theo taps the screen. "Here— 'We cannot allow extraction. We can only permit examination.' They mean everything has to stay on site."

Andrew nods. "Then we'll take the lab to them."

They design mobile clean labs that are fully sealed, and each unit is certified for sterile containment to ensure genetic material never leaves the country. In-depth and recurring testing will be done in cooperation with a French lab already on board.

Theo grins faintly. "I can't believe we just negotiated international microbiology diplomacy."

Meera smiles. "You make it sound almost glamorous."

Just as progress seems certain, the final and most unexpected challenge emerges—the local custodians of the cemeteries. Groundskeepers, clergy, and caretakers hold no formal authority over research approvals, but their cooperation is everything. The government's permit grants access; the custodians grant acceptance. A single complaint could be enough to stall or even revoke the authorization.

In Colleville-sur-Mer, they learn of a man named Gérard who has tended the American cemetery for forty years. His word carries weight with both local officials and visiting families. Emails to him go unanswered, and he declines a virtual meeting. "If they want to touch the soil," he tells the liaison, "they can look me in the eye first."

This creates a new hurdle. Travel requests must be submitted. Meera and Theo are willing, but Dell Children's, still wary after the last board meeting, will only approve travel for one. "We will not authorize a diplomatic expedition," Harold writes in his reply. "Send your lead."

Andrew volunteers. He knows the data best, and he understands the stakes. The coalition agrees.

Andrew departs Austin at 6:15 p.m. on a transatlantic flight routed through Dallas and then Paris. By the time he lands at Charles de Gaulle, bleary-eyed and rumpled, nearly twelve hours have passed. A regional train from Gare Saint-Lazare takes him to Bayeux, and from there, he rents a compact Peugeot that smells faintly of lavender and diesel. The drive to Colleville-sur-Mer winds through hedgerows and distant church steeples. By the time he reaches the coast, it's mid-afternoon, just within the cemetery's visiting hours. Altogether, it has taken him nearly eighteen hours in transit to reach this quiet field of memory.

Gérard is skeptical from the moment Andrew arrives. The groundskeeper meets him at the edge of the gravel path, weathered and silent, his eyes wary under a gray flat cap. They walk together between rows of white crosses, saying little at first. When they reach a tall cedar tree at the center of the cemetery, Gérard finally stops.

"You want to dig here," he says. "You want to ask the ground to speak."

Andrew nods. "Only in places away from the graves. Discreet, reversible. We've already agreed not to take any material away. The French Ministry, the VA, the consulates... they've all approved."

Gérard says nothing for a long time. The wind moves between the rows.

"They approved what is easy to approve. But this... This is memory. Not yours. Not mine. Theirs," Gérard offers while carrying his gaze to the rows of headstones and flowers.

Andrew explains again what they've seen in the soil, the microbial gaps, and the epigenetic signals. He tells Gérard they will not disturb; they want to understand. To honor legacy through knowledge while preserving the soil, headstones, and those fallen.

Still, Gérard says little. He offers no blessing, no refusal. Just a small gesture toward the crosses.

"These are more than names," he finally says. "They are promises. Don't dig unless you understand what it means to disturb that memory."

Andrew bows slightly, not sure whether the meeting is over. Silently, Gérard turns with a gesture and walks him back in silence.

They wait another four weeks before receiving his letter of approval. It contains no formal letterhead. Just a short note written with a fountain pen that reads, "If the soil speaks, I hope it says something kind."

With Gérard's letter in hand, the team turns next to their respective institutions. Formal travel plans, equipment procurement, and international permissions must now be underwritten. Andrew and Theo both approach Dell Children's, navigating parallel channels through research administration and clinical leadership. Meera circles back to her ethics board in Hyderabad. All three make the case with renewed urgency. The groundwork has been laid. The permissions are real. The questions are bigger than ever.

This time, they find approval. Meera's hospital agrees to fund a portion of the laboratory supplies and travel, contingent upon updates and a final report. Dell Children's, though cautious, agrees to support both Andrew and Theo. Andrew receives funding for participation and travel, while Theo secures equipment support and shared departmental resources. Each institution imposes its own layers of reporting and oversight, but the green lights arrive nonetheless. The expedition becomes real.

Their small team comprises the three research leads, five technicians, two portable labs, and clearance for limited core sampling in predefined grid zones. They make their base in Bayeux, a town known for its medieval tapestry and cobbled charm. The hotel is modest. It's wooden shutters, iron balconies, and the scent of espresso and morning rain drifting through the halls. Meera walks the stone streets at dusk, gathering her thoughts. Theo finds a quiet spot in the now-empty breakfast room to revise the checklist one last time. Andrew, jet-lagged but steady, pores over coordinates and mapping data.

After a full night of rest, they regroup in the hotel's gravel courtyard, load the portable labs into two rental vans, and make the winding drive to the coast. As they approach Colleville-sur-Mer, the terrain flattens and the sea draws near. Wind bends the tall grass sideways. The road narrows.

Then, the cemetery emerges.

It stretches before them under a heavy gray sky, white crosses in perfect rows, grass too green to be accidental. The stillness is absolute. A reverent hush holds the grounds, broken only by the soft rustle of wind and the distant gulls. Here, the dead do not rest in obscurity. They lie in symmetry, in memory, in collective solemnity.

Theo crouches near the first site, assembling the bore sampler. Andrew records coordinates. Meera watches the horizon. The air carries salt and silence.

She thinks of her grandfather's stories. Stories of the return from war, of how the land remembers what we let go. She remembers the forests of her childhood, the sacred groves that pulsed with unseen inheritance. Here, far from home, that same hush lingers. Meera kneels and touches the soil with connection, whispering an apology.

"We are here to listen, to observe with care and respect."

Behind her, one of the technicians, Julia, a soil microbiologist from Utrecht, carefully unpacks sterile vials and gloves. She adjusts her scarf against the wind and murmurs, "My great-grandfather is buried not far from here, in a cemetery across the border. I never met him, but this..." Her words trail off for a moment. "It feels like meeting him."

Another technician, Alain, a French forensic specialist, speaks with a hushed accent. "These crosses, they stand like sentinels, but what lies beneath is not silent. The land has absorbed their memory."

They drill carefully, avoiding root systems and memorial structures. Soil samples are labeled, logged, and sealed. The team works methodically, recording GPS coordinates, photographing each core sample site, and logging initial soil color, consistency, and scent. Alain calls out moisture readings, while Julia notes the presence of mycorrhizal networks, thick and fibrous in some cores and nearly absent in others.

Still, the weight of place is never far. Each step between the rows feels like trespass. The ground is hallowed, historically, emotionally, and in ways that can be felt as much as understood. At one point, Theo stops mid-measurement and whispers, "I feel like we're digging into silence."

Alain pauses, hands muddy. "My uncle is buried in Normandy. Not here, but close. He was nineteen." His voice falters, and he looks away, blinking rapidly. The auger slips slightly in his hand. He crouches, ostensibly to adjust the sampling kit, but his shoulders curl inward, and for a moment, he doesn't move.

"I used to think about what he might've looked like," he murmurs, barely audible. "My grandmother never spoke of him. It was too much."

Julia sets a hand on his back, a gesture of comfort, trying to connect, to see him, to witness his grief and stand with him in it. Her presence is quiet and unwavering. For a few long moments, she says nothing, just lets her hand rest between his shoulders. Alain wipes his cheek with his sleeve, then steadies himself.

"Sorry," he says. "It just... It catches you off guard. Being here."

Julia withdraws her hand gently from Alain's back, pressing it instead to her own chest, voice barely audible. "I didn't think it would feel this personal. I thought the science would protect us from that."

Meera replies gently, "Maybe the science doesn't protect us. Maybe it's how we bear witness."

They rotate teams every hour, partly to prevent fatigue, but also to give each person a moment to step back and breathe, to acknowledge what they are walking through. Andrew joins one of the technicians in silence, carefully handing over sample labels. When the auger sticks in a dense patch of clay, he kneels beside it and loosens the earth by hand, as if unwilling to force it.

The silence in the cemetery hums with presence. Every tool they use, every vial they seal, becomes a pact. An act of listening that honors the place and those buried there.

At first, the data returns as expected. Standard soil profiles, with variables in moisture levels, fungal density, and carbon distribution. No anomalies. Just the slow rhythm of controlled sampling.

Then, small surprises begin to surface. Trace levels of unusual bacterial colonies. Subtle shifts in mineral concentration bands. Patterns that suggest long-term organic degradation occurring in ways that don't follow typical decay curves. It's like faint echoes of a song remembered from childhood.

Then, the DNA traces begin to emerge.

Not intact genomes or even full profiles. Just whispers. Degraded mitochondrial fragments, epigenetic tags, and residual biological signatures cling to the biome. Some samples contain sequences that match 1940s

European polymorphisms. Others are more ambiguous. Traces that don't correspond to modern populations but suggest long-dead variance still echoing in the microbiota.

Theo stares at the data. "Being here… it's different," he says quietly.

Julia rests a hand on his shoulder. "It's not the numbers, is it? It's knowing who they belonged to."

The day is long and layered. Each team works from a detailed map of pre-approved zones, dividing the cemetery grid into sectors by nationality and burial depth. They extract three to five samples at each site, including topsoil, mid-core, and sub-core. The portable labs hum in the background, their chilled compartments slowly filling with vials sealed in triplicate. Julia oversees microbial plating protocols, Alain records environmental variables with a handheld spectrometer, and Theo coordinates timestamps with the metadata log.

By mid-afternoon, over sixty samples have been collected. Some are dense with root networks, others strangely barren. Soil from the German section carries a sharper metallic scent, while the American plots seem darker and thicker. Each technician works with careful hands and quiet solidarity.

They run replication sequences through the night, alert to every anomaly. One soil sample shows a faint recurrence of a microRNA family long suppressed by modern conditions. Another, taken near a German soldier's marker, carries methylation patterns that mirror stress-response signatures found in mid-century tissue samples archived in Berlin.

"It looks like a re-emergence," Theo says. Conditions aligning just enough to let the pattern surface again."

Andrew studies the graph. "So, the soil chemistry is reproducing the same stress environment that produced those signatures in the first place."

Theo nods. "Exactly. Environment echoing environment."

Later that night, long after the data had been logged and the final centrifuge had slowed, the team stepped outside the hotel together. The air was cool and moist, and the streets of Bayeux were hushed beneath amber streetlamps. Meera walked a few paces ahead, drawn toward a small courtyard garden behind the hotel. The others followed.

There, beneath a moon partially veiled by clouds, Meera kneels and presses her palm against the damp earth. Her skin tingles at the contact. The soil is cool, alive in ways the eye can't see. The others stand nearby, silent. No one needs to speak.

Her thoughts move through generations of conflict and repair, cycles of loss, decomposition, and return. The ground beneath her holds the molecular remains of those histories, layered and reactive, the biological record of human disturbance. The earth retains that archive.

The dead do not remain. They transform, diffusing through microbial pathways, mineral bonds, and biochemical exchange.

What once seemed like memory is a mechanism of genetic fragments interacting with the environment.

Andrew finds a bench just off the courtyard path, its wrought-iron frame cold beneath him. He sits slowly, as if the weight of the day still presses on him. The lamp above flickers once, then steadies. Meera and Theo sit nearby on the edge of the stone planter, neither speaking. For a long moment, they just breathe. They are aware of the night, the earth, and the work they've dared to do.

The Normandy soil glows in their vials, under microscopes, on laminated printouts pinned to the mobile lab walls. The light reveals what history leaves behind, an ongoing exchange between what was lost and what endures. The fallen are part of the pattern now, their remnants active within the living field.

CHAPTER 13
CARRIED HOME IN SILENCE

The team arrives home in waves, each crossing continents under different skies, carrying with them the weight of what they've seen and touched. The return flights are quiet, filled with unread books and half-finished notes, their bodies fatigued from long hours and compressed timelines. Normandy had offered them only a brief window. Seventy-two hours of sampling, cross-referencing, logging, and analysis. Now, the real work begins.

By the time Meera reaches her apartment, the city is deep in sleep. The streets outside are slick with rain, reflecting yellow streetlamps in broken puddles. She keys the door open quietly, not bothering to turn on the lights. Inside, the silence greets her like an old friend. Her bags drop to the floor with a dull thud. Shoes off. Hair unpinned. She moves through the motions as if underwater.

Theo and Andrew arrive home in Austin several hours apart, each on separate flights arranged through different hospital travel channels. Andrew stayed an extra day to finalize archival documentation with the French consulate, while Theo traveled back with the equipment crates to ensure their safe transfer.

Theo's arrival back in Austin is abrupt. When he walks into his apartment, he doesn't bother with lights or luggage. He collapses face-down on the couch. His laptop is still powered in sleep mode, now placed hurriedly on the coffee table, notes and protein bars scattered to make room for it. He holds on to consciousness just long enough to plug in his phone and scribble a reminder to upload the data the next morning.

Andrew returns to Austin the following day. His flight lands just after dusk, and the terminal feels too bright, too busy after the solemn quiet of Normandy. Sonia waits just beyond the security barrier, holding a to-go coffee in one hand and scanning the arriving passengers with impatient eyes. When she spots him, her face lights up, but she tempers it quickly, recognizing the wear etched into his posture.

"You're really back," she says softly, handing him a coffee. "You look like you haven't slept in a week."

"I feel like I haven't," Andrew replies with a wan smile. "And we barely got the last samples logged before we had to pack it all up."

Sonia asks about the trip on the drive home, about Normandy, the data, and what they found. Andrew answers in short phrases, his voice distant. He doesn't mean to evade the conversation; he's just depleted emotionally and physically.

Once inside the house, he drops his bag just inside the door and leaves it there. Sonia watches him for a moment, then silently makes tea in the kitchen while Andrew takes a long shower. He eats a little, writes a few notes by hand in his notebook, and then sits in the living room with the lights off.

The work will begin soon, but stillness is the only thing he can manage for now.

Meera, Theo, and Andrew don't speak about the samples at first. For twelve hours, they go silent. No calls, messages, or lab reports. Each of them needs the time to decompress, sleep, and reacclimate to the lives and time zones they left behind. Jet lag winds through their limbs like a fog, and even the thought of reopening the project feels momentarily impossible. They reengage only after this recovery space, one by one, Andrew coming in last.

When they finally reconnect, it's not to marvel at what they found. They coordinate timelines, processing queues, which lab gets first access, and how the data is to be partitioned, catalogued, and secured. Theo had already started organizing everything, his spreadsheet color-coded with tabs for sample origin, sequencing priority, and lab routing.

"Okay," Theo says as the screen loads their first call, his voice quick and bright, "I've got everything color-coded and cross-tabbed. Sample origin, sequencing priority, lab routing, you name it. Also…"

"Hold on," Meera interrupts, rubbing her eyes. "What time is it again?"

"Too early in the day for this nonsense," Andrew adds with a yawn. "How are you this awake?"

"I brought back Turkish coffee," Theo declares. "It's rocket fuel. I haven't blinked since Tuesday."

There's a brief silence, then Andrew groans. "Oh, damn! That explains everything."

"Are you vibrating?" Meera teases. "Do I hear drumming?"

Theo grins into the camera. "Steering wheel makes an excellent desk."

"You're not in a car, are you?" Andrew says.

"No, but I was, and I could still coordinate batch uploads. That's dedication."

Meera chuckles. "Or madness."

"Why not both?" Theo says brightly.

The banter settles them, each in their own windowed box, thousands of miles apart, but suddenly reconnected. The rhythm of scientific discipline resumes, steady and methodical. And yes, slightly caffeinated.

Andrew groans faintly in the background, still not fully adjusted. Meera chuckles but doesn't question it. Theo's energy, unfiltered and slightly manic, keeps the wheels turning while the rest of them catch up. The rhythm of scientific discipline resumes, steady and methodical, and to the sound of Theo drumming… now on his desk.

Within forty-eight hours, they're back in rhythm. The portable lab files are uploaded, redundancies checked, and encrypted servers humming to life. Meera takes on the sample indexing with the same clinical clarity she used in

France. Her voice crisp over the transcontinental calls. Andrew begins the first wave of microbial drift modeling, while Theo sets up the sequencing queue, batch by painstaking batch.

The results will take weeks, maybe months. But the signal—the whisper in the soil—they all heard it. Now they must prove it.

Meera sets the sequencing calendar, building in weekly review checkpoints and alternating analysis windows between Hyderabad and Austin. Theo maintains the master spreadsheet, highlighting emerging anomalies in orange and flagging low-yield samples in gray. Andrew's modeling interface grows with each passing day, a quiet constellation of data points mapping the unseen legacy beneath Normandy.

Every morning, new comparisons are made. DNA fragment length is compared to soil density, microbial colony composition is compared to historical burial records, and epigenetic tags are compared to geographic markers. The signal sharpens by degrees, whisper by whisper.

They live in the liminal space between certainty and implication. Between what the data shows and what it dares to mean.

Reports begin arriving from the partner labs, labs they'd leaned on in earlier phases of the research: Camila's team in São Paulo, the Japanese soil chemistry lab in Osaka, and the small but tenacious genetic unit in Rotterdam. Each group received a segment of the Normandy soil analysis, which was anonymized and randomized. Each group has direct access to the labs in France for continued monitoring and testing.

Some results return murky, degraded signals and inconclusive banding. Camila reports high organic noise in several samples due to storm-soaked soil. While others, particularly those pulled from shaded glades along the cemetery perimeter, yield something more.

Something more like structures. Not intact genomes. Nonetheless, there are distinctive patterns. The presence of nucleotide scaffolding. Unlinked fragments and base pair residues that shouldn't persist after seventy-five years. The labs call them precursors, environmental building blocks that show clear statistical clustering near the burial zones.

"The fragments are coherent even though they aren't viable in a biological sense," the report from Rotterdam clarifies. "That coherence is the anomaly."

As the team begins to chart the returns, a pattern emerges. Samples closest to individual gravesites hold higher concentrations of these remnants. Control samples from walkways and untouched forest perimeters show far less.

The data is still fragmentary, but it coheres. Theo overlays burial dates, Meera compares soil stratification patterns, and Andrew runs multivariate regression on burial density versus molecular residue.

Then comes the turning point. The statistical signal reaches relevance. More than possibility, it's probability.

They stare at the graphs, the trend lines, the residue maps. Slowly, the implication dawns. The earth may carry trace DNA residue in ways no one has ever dared to measure.

It's the question they've been circling for weeks, one they pushed aside until the evidence forced it back. Now that correlation is established, meaning becomes unavoidable.

Theo leans back in his chair during one exchange and says what they've all been thinking. "Okay. Say this is real. Say the earth really does archive us. Call it genetic scaffolds, environmental echoes, or whatever this is. How does that help the living? How do we connect this to anomaly rates, birth defects, or resilience?"

Meera nods slowly, her voice confident. "It's not about reanimating the dead or reconstructing anyone's identity. It's about understanding environmental influence and the silent undercurrents. These fragments we're seeing might not be viable for replication, but they're still chemically and structurally active. They persist in ways we never accounted for."

Meera continues, "Epigenetics is sensitive. It's not always about changing DNA. It's about regulating it. Environmental factors can upregulate or silence genes, especially in developing embryos. One example people often relate to is how a mother's nutrition or stress during pregnancy can impact the child's long-term health. The mother's health does not change their genes but alters how they are expressed. This is the same, except that the land responds with precision. Rather than altering DNA itself, it regulates its activity."

She continues, "If these genetic fragments persist in the soil long enough, they might influence the microbial environment around early human development. They might shape chemical exposures or trigger gene activation or suppression subtly and consistently over time, not causing mutations but steering development."

She gestures toward the shared screen, where the maps are layered with dots and colors. "So, if the soil carries historical patterns, then yes, proximity to certain legacies might confer risk. Or protection. These are echoes of presence, diffused into biology. I think we're measuring more than contamination. We might be looking at the long tail of influence, inherited through place."

Andrew rubs his temples, his voice deliberate. "Let's bring this back to where it started. The defect clusters we've seen are not abstract. They're babies in NICUs, kids who never made it home. What if those clusters aren't random at all? What if proximity to historical burial zones creates persistent environmental fields? Specifically, mass graves, wartime cemeteries, or sites soaked in biological loss. Not functional DNA, but a residue. Ghost signals. And those signals shape what comes next."

Theo whistles softly. "Genetic weather. A microclimate of influence."

"Exactly," Meera says. "If we can model that influence or understand what degrades and persists, then we might be able to predict areas of elevated risk. Else, we'll find regions where resilience is mysteriously high."

Andrew nods. "From there, we will introduce interventions. Soil buffering. Microbial countermeasures. Even public health zoning. If we know where the residuals linger, we may be able to preempt environmental epigenetic disruption. We might save children from patterns they never chose."

The team goes momentarily quiet. It's time to begin combining the theory and the responsibility. They've spent months confirming that the signal exists. Now comes the question they've been circling since the beginning: can it be changed?

Meera speaks first. "I've been modeling potential field sites for months. There's a burial ground on the outskirts of Hyderabad. It's revered and ancient. No embalming. No stone vaults. Just soil."

She hesitates, weighing her words. "It's precisely because it's a burial ground that it matters. We already know biological scaffolding persists in soils touched by the dead. What we've agreed needs to be identified next is whether the signal is static or responsive."

Theo frowns slightly. "So, you're saying we introduce new material to see if the existing signature reacts?"

"Exactly," Meera says. "Think of it like tuning a signal. We're observing how legacy and enrichment interact. Introducing healthy microbial buffers—native, enriched soil strains—will show us whether the memory holds, blends, or changes."

Andrew asks, "Wouldn't enrichment reduce what we're trying to study?"

"Clarify," she says. "Refine the signal. If the legacy material holds strong, we'll see it clearly. If it's malleable, we'll see that too. We're not looking to erase the presence. We're studying how it behaves in a biologically dynamic system. That's the only way we begin to understand its impact and how to mitigate it in places where that legacy is…" She pauses for a moment, looking for the right word. "deficient and potentially hurting children. If we could introduce enriched microbial material, a form of soil buffering treatment, we might be able to measure how the biome changes. Whether the legacy signal weakens or strengthens."

Theo's eyebrows lift, realizing what she's just suggested. "Wait. You want to test on sacred ground?"

"It's not an excavation. It's surface-level enrichment. Observational," Meera replies. "But yes, it's near a place people hold sacred. I'll handle it with care."

Andrew's voice carries a note of caution. "You're sure you want to be the first to propose this?"

"Someone has to start the controls," she replies. "If we're right about the mechanism, the model needs field confirmation. It's merely replication."

Undeterred, she prepares the documentation meticulously, anticipating the questions before they arrive. Her hospital's research board is the first step. She presents the proposal as an observational study with ecological and public health implications, emphasizing its non-invasive approach. She outlines the enrichment method as microbial infusion via topsoil misting, using strains native to the region. No digging. No soil removal. Just a gentle nudge to see what shifts.

The board listens. Some members are intrigued; others are hesitant. One asks whether the soil's history has been adequately respected. Another worries aloud about optics, about how this might look in the media. Meera answers with calm, steady resolve, presenting the scientific rationale and the spiritual caution she's built into the plan. The board deliberates for two days before granting conditional approval, requiring biweekly updates and complete transparency with community stakeholders.

Next comes the local municipal authority. Here, the process is slower and more bureaucratic. Forms are misfiled, and emails go unanswered. A clerical error sends the proposal to the parks department instead of the environmental bureau. Meera resubmits, calls offices directly, and speaks with advisors late into the evening. It takes over a week just to get it onto the right desk.

Then, without notice, it leaks. A minor government employee forwards the proposal to a local preservation group. Within forty-eight hours, it's circulating on WhatsApp and Twitter under the headline: "Scientist Plans to Experiment on Burial Ground."

What begins as curiosity quickly becomes anger.

A protest erupts outside the university gates the following morning. Initially, the crowd is small, primarily students and elders from nearby neighborhoods, but it swells by noon. Men in saffron robes chant beneath hand-painted banners. Women arrive bearing garlands and folded prayer cloths. Some carry photographs of ancestors buried at the site, holding them like shields. One protester is carrying a sign that reads, "Our ancestors are not your laboratory." Others pass out flyers quoting spiritual texts about the sanctity of rest. There's even a flyer about how soil remembers what people try to forget.

Seeing that last one show up on social media, Theo frowns and turns his phone toward the camera during their video call. "That's your language," he says to Meera. "They're quoting your theory back at you."

Meera's expression tightens. "Then one of our drafts got out."

No one speaks for a moment. They all know what that means.

Meera stared at the line again through someone else's framing: "The soil remembers what people try to forget." It was almost word-for-word from her initial proposal draft; a line she'd used to describe residual microbial inheritance. Yet here, in bold print on a flyer handed out by protesters, it had transformed into a warning or an accusation.

"It's been twisted," she said quietly. "They've taken something observational and made it sacred."

Theo agreed. "That's the problem with ideas once they're released. They stop belonging to us."

Outside, the chanting grew louder: "Do not desecrate what protects us." "Leave the soil to silence, not science." "The body may decay, but the spirit lives in the ground."

Inside, the team exchanged uneasy glances, watching this unfold in real time. They had predicted this exact scenario. Words are lifted from their research and turned against them in a public square. What was once an academic metaphor had become a spiritual rallying cry. The line that had helped Meera frame the persistence of molecular trace had now become proof, in the protestors' eyes, that she was attempting to violate sacred memory.

"It's the risk of visibility," Andrew said. "Every time we tried to publish something earlier, we worried it would be misunderstood."

Meera nodded. "It moved beyond misunderstanding. It has become weaponized."

Theo ran a hand through his hair. "We spent all that time trying to make it accessible, and now it's been taken completely out of context."

Local media arrive. Reporters push microphones toward anyone willing to speak. One woman holds up a small jar of earth from the site and sobs. Another, a teenage boy in a school uniform, recites a poem he wrote the night before. Meera watches from her office while Andrew and Theo observe from their homes. Her name is on the banners now.

Then a priest steps forward, flanked by followers in crisp white dhotis and long strands of rudraksha beads. He speaks with authority, his voice clear even without amplification.

"She seeks to disturb the souls of the dead," he says. "To test and probe what is meant to be sacred. Science has its place. Just not here. Not on consecrated ground."

He lifts a hand to the sky. "You do not plant on memory," he says. "You do not till grief."

Meera listens in silence with her hands folded in front of her. Elsewhere, the hospital's associate dean of research receives an emergency call. By dusk, the proposal is suspended pending further review.

The next day, the hospital's ethics committee at Dell Children's requests a full briefing from Andrew and Theo. The media attention has raised concerns about institutional alignment, liability, and the perception of involvement. A subcommittee is convened via video call to review the study's objectives and the language used in early publications.

"I'm not saying your science is unsound," one board member says, "but when public understanding diverges this dramatically, it's no longer just about results. It's about reputation."

Theo tries to explain the intent behind the terminology. Andrew reemphasizes the potential for long-term health applications, but the questions come faster than answers. Who owns the data? How are communities being consulted? What mechanisms are in place to prevent spiritual or cultural transgressions?

Meanwhile, Meera requests an audience with the associate dean. She dresses in muted colors, a sign of both respect and caution, and carries a revised version of her proposal under one arm. This time, she brings letters of support from colleagues, revised language free of metaphor, and a proposed partnership with a local cultural liaison to help bridge the divide between science and sentiment.

The dean receives her with reserved politeness, motioning to a chair opposite his desk. Outside, students walk past the window in loose knots, some still carrying protest signs. Meera waits until he sets aside his phone.

"I'd like to request a second review," she says simply.

He studies her for a long moment. Then he nods. "You'll have it. But tread carefully. The ground you're standing on isn't just sacred. It's shifting."

CHAPTER 14
EDGE OF CONSENT

A week has passed since the protests. The echo of chants still lingers in Meera's mind, but today, her focus narrows to the meeting ahead. She's pacing her office, waving a manila folder in her hand like a wand while murmuring something under her breath. Andrew and Theo watch silently for a moment through their shared video connection while she's working it out. The three have continued their regular meetings to keep research analysis progressing while they navigate their support and funding concerns.

"You're going to wear a hole in the floor," Theo says, spinning slightly in his chair. "Though I suppose if the building collapses, we'll get some interesting sediment layers to test."

Meera stops pacing just long enough to shoot him a look, half-annoyed, half-grateful. "You know this could go either way, right?"

Andrew lays down his tablet, sensing the gravity beneath her words. "He's a challenging audience, but you've got something undeniable. Those letters have peer-reviewed backing from a global network of researchers. That means something."

Meera nods and clutches the folder closer to her chest. "They didn't just express support. They're offering funding, lab space, and field access.

Even their own datasets. They all say that the work has to continue, and it has to be us."

Theo raises an eyebrow. "Wow, actual money? So, we're finally moving up from ramen-tier science?"

"Speak for yourself," Meera says dryly. "I happen to like instant noodles."

"Sure, but only because you haven't lived the horror of Theo's kitchen experiments," Andrew adds. "Last week, he tried to make protein bars out of freeze-dried lentils and peanut butter."

"Innovation through desperation," Theo says, undeterred. "You can thank me when I patent them."

Meera smiles despite herself, then glances down at the folder again. Inside are letters from Japan, Brazil, South Africa, and the Netherlands. Some are formal, others handwritten. All express urgency. They acknowledge the backlash surrounding the burial site proposal and the fear that it might derail the very research the world is starting to notice.

"They believe in us," she says softly. "Even with the controversy. Maybe because of it."

Andrew stands and walks contemplatively away from the camera. "Then bring that into the room with you. Bring more than the folder, bring the belief. If the dean sees that the world is watching, maybe he'll stop acting like it's just our mess to clean up."

She takes a breath. A long, full one. Then nods. "Alright. Time to face the music. Or at least the string section."

"Play it in a minor key," Theo says, offering a small bow. "For dramatic effect."

"Knock 'em dead," Andrew adds, more seriously.

She closes the connection and exits toward the administrative wing, shoulders back and folder in hand. Behind her, the door clicks shut, and for a moment, the hallway is still.

Associate Dean Harish Malhotra sits behind a wide desk that somehow feels too formal for the government hospital. Books on genetics and ethics fill the shelves behind him while his eyes remain fixed on Meera. He gestures for her to sit.

"Dr. Rao," he begins, folding his hands together. "I've read the revised proposal. I've also read every article, letter, and op-ed that's crossed my desk in the past week. Some from colleagues. Some from strangers. One from a priest..." He pauses, scanning the tablet on his desk, then reads aloud with dry precision, "who called you an 'architect of desecration.'"

Meera doesn't flinch. "And twenty-three letters from researchers urging the science to continue. Including labs offering to help fund the work themselves."

"Yes," he says slowly. "They're impressive. Passionate. This goes beyond science alone. You proposed soil sampling near a sacred burial site. That invites not only scientific scrutiny, but also public and political enquiry."

She opens the folder and slides the stack of letters forward. "They offer more than their passion. They bring credibility. Experts in virology, soil genomics, and epigenetics have already joined the collaboration. We aim to preserve the graves while studying what time leaves behind in the soil."

"A poetic way to describe it," Harish replies, brows lifting.

"It's accurate," Meera says. "We know genetic drift is happening. We've found patterns, decay points, and geographic clusters. What's happening in these soils may be the missing link. We're seeing inherited absence in children whose families have no known genetic history of illness, and we believe environmental transfer is at play."

"And what of the burial ground?"

"It isn't about the dead. It's about what remains. It's about under-standing how past generations might be affecting the current one through microbiotic or chemical traces. We've been careful. We've never suggested excavation, only enrichment tracking."

Dean Malhotra steeples his fingers. "You've become the face of this controversy, Meera. The local news is circling. There are murmurs in Parliament. If I sign off, and this doesn't go well..."

"Then you'll face questions," Meera finishes. "Publicly. Maybe profes-sionally. I understand what I'm asking. However, standing still signals a decision just as clearly, one that accelerates degradation through inaction."

He stares at her for a long moment. Then he picks up one of the letters on Dutch letterhead, neat handwriting, and a seal from Utrecht University.

"I recognize this name. I worked with van der Kooi on a rare pathogen case fifteen years ago. Brilliant man. Prickly, but honest."

He sets the letter down, then opens a drawer and pulls out the stamped approval sheet.

"I'm signing this against my better judgment," he says, pen poised. "You'd better be right about this. If this becomes another scandal, I'll lose the ability to shield you next time, ...or myself."

"Understood," Meera says quietly.

He signs.

"Get to work, Dr. Rao."

She nods, holding the folder a little tighter as she walks out. This time, there is no echo of protest in her ears. There is only the sound of progress stirring at the edges.

Outside the office, Meera doesn't return to her lab immediately. Instead, she steps into the courtyard just beyond the administrative wing. The sun is harsh on the stone, but the silence is welcome. She settles onto a shaded bench and opens the folder again, though she no longer reads the letters. She knows their contents by heart.

Since returning from Normandy, the science has evolved, while, at the same time, so has the resistance. France had offered more than genetic fragments; it revealed a working model of how legacy DNA, though no longer viable for replication, might still shape the living. Meera had seen the influence in the soil. Genetic echoes that seeded microbial shifts, cascades of biological expression through them. The implications had been breathtaking and unsettling. Still, applying that model back home proved more complicated.

Then came the burial site outside Hyderabad. The backlash was swift. A proposal meant to heal became framed as harm. Now, with a significant cost, this has received approval.

She traces her finger over the edge of the folder. Access to the original site remains blocked for now due to public pressure. Still, the science continues. The model for soil buffering, using enriched microbial material at burial boundaries, remains viable. The team now searches for a new location that shares similar geological and cultural conditions and where oversight and trust can thrive.

Trust.

She breathes in deeply, the air thick with heat and old jasmine. It will take delicate planning, rebuilding rapport with local officials, and reframing the study's purpose. They'll have to invite in more voices, like cultural historians or spiritual advisors. And maybe that's a good thing. Perhaps it forces them to disregard this as pure science and treat the work more as a story.

Because what they're testing isn't just microbial enrichment. It's the echo of everything once rooted here, still vibrating beneath their feet. Moreover, it's the possibility that the ground absorbs every decision they make.

Dell Children's Medical Center's conference room is full, restless, expectant, and lined with authority. Andrew sits to the left of the projection screen, Theo beside him, both physically present and fully exposed beneath the room's scrutiny. They are surrounded by a semicircle of department heads, two senior ethicists, and the president of the hospital, Dr. Lauren Channing. This isn't an ordinary meeting. It's a reckoning. Their research has drawn global attention, and with it comes local scrutiny. News coverage of the overseas protests has linked the hospital's name to the controversy, raising questions of oversight and reputation. What unfolds here will determine whether the hospital remains a partner in the effort or distances itself completely. Around the room, clipboards rest on crossed knees, pens hover over margins, and every eye is fixed on the two men who now represent a science that dares to reach beneath the surface, literally and ethically.

The air is thick with anticipation and doubt.

"Let's get to it," Dr. Channing says, tapping her pen once against her notepad. "We've all read the research summary and the letters of support. What we need to understand now is broader than just the science. Dr. Turbin, the first question on everyone's mind is who owns this data?"

Andrew doesn't hesitate. "The data is stewarded by a global consortium, with institutional review boards in every participating country. Our team does not claim exclusive ownership. Raw data is anonymized and housed on mirrored servers governed by a shared access protocol. Our role is analysis, not possession."

"And what of the families for the children?" asks Dr. Patel, chair of neonatology. "What role do they have in consent?"

"We've implemented tiered opt-in models at every site," Theo explains. "We've engaged parent advocacy groups in the design of those forms. In Austin alone, we held three listening sessions before rollout. We're co-creating the terms, not just collecting samples."

A rustle of murmured approval passes through the room.

Dr. Abernathy, the chair of pediatric ethics, leans forward, voice probing. "You've addressed informed consent and cultural consultation, but how are you managing the emotional landscape this research intersects? You're talking about burial grounds, ancestral remains, and legacy trauma. Are mental health professionals part of your outreach teams?"

"Yes," Andrew replies. "We've brought in pediatric psychologists and grief counselors during preliminary discussions, and we're integrating trauma-informed practices into every level of community interaction. We aim to understand how history imprints itself chemically and socially. The aim is to acknowledge the grief and work within the cultural rituals."

"What about political entanglements?" asks Dr. Willis from pathology. "Once governments get involved, especially internationally, how do you safeguard the science?"

Theo replies, "That's already happening. Instead of resisting it, we're creating shared oversight agreements. When possible, we partner with both public institutions and NGOs, ensuring that no single entity, whether governmental or academic, controls the narrative. We have to model transparency in every layer."

Dr. Channing taps her pen again. "You're essentially asking us to become stewards of ethical unknowns. This reaches beyond hospital research. It's civil, cultural, even existential."

"That's true," Andrew says. "But the alternative is worse. If we shy away now, someone else will take this work underground. Less scrutiny, less care. We believe it should remain in the light."

This time, the nods are slower and heavier. The room seems to be absorbing the responsibility suggested by this proposal. Somehow, it feels more like an acknowledgment than any kind of approval.

"Then let's talk about the land," says one of the ethics committee members. "How are local communities being consulted before you introduce enriched materials? Especially in proximity to culturally sensitive sites?"

Andrew exhales. "That part is harder. We've just lost access to one such site in India after a public backlash. Meera, Dr. Rao, is working directly with religious scholars and local governance councils to identify new partners. We've also begun assembling a cultural advisory board composed of historians, spiritual leaders, and Indigenous scientists."

Theo looks at Andrew and then at Dr. Channing. "We know this project doesn't just operate in the realm of molecules. It touches memory, legacy, and grief. That means we move only with full consent and cultural alignment."

Dr. Channing nods slowly. "What's the safeguard if someone says no?"

"Then the answer is no," Andrew says plainly. "Our model is designed to pause or pivot. Full transparency. No back doors. No workarounds."

Silence follows. Then one of the ethics advisors speaks, softer than the rest. "You're treating soil as if it carries identity. I think that's what makes this both beautiful and dangerous."

Theo smiles faintly. "Exactly."

Dr. Channing taps her pen again; however, this time it's more thoughtful than sharp. "You have my support. But let me be clear; this buys you credibility, not immunity. The moment you lose community trust, this stops."

Andrew nods. "We understand."

"Then go forward, and tread carefully."

The meeting ends with quiet nods, pens capping, and a lingering weight in the air that feels like a warning and a welcome. They have permission now and all the responsibilities that come with it.

Three days later, the core coalition of researchers assembles again. This time on a video call that spans six different time zones. Faces blink to life on the screen: Dr. Lotte van Dalen from Utrecht, Camila Rocha and Dr. Mariana Reis from São Paulo, Professor Kaoru Watanabe and Dr.

Satoshi Nishida from Japan, and Dr. Themba Mokoena from Cape Town. Meera joins from Hyderabad, with Andrew and Theo seated together in Austin. The mood is more measured than their last meeting, less celebratory and more surgical.

"We've all read the fallout," Camila begins without preamble. Her voice is to the point and clipped. "The protest in Hyderabad and the parliamentary comments. I assume the local approval was re-secured?"

"It was," Meera confirms, adjusting her headset. "Just barely. However, we've lost access to the original site."

"That might be a blessing in disguise," Themba says. "It's pushed the conversation forward. We're no longer just talking about environmental influence; we're now accountable for cultural legacy."

Mariana nods. "That's where we stumbled. The science was strong, but the framing failed. We made the language too clinical, too detached. Burial soil carries deep meaning for the communities that live near it. We have to begin every proposal with that truth."

Theo stares straight ahead, camera slightly off-angle. "We've begun compiling an internal protocol with ethics checkpoints before any soil work near human remains. More than IRB clearance, local consultations, language audits, and spiritual liaisons."

"Those measures should be published," Satoshi adds. "If we're serious about responsible science, we model it openly. Let others hold us to it."

Andrew shares a screen showing excerpts from two recent peer-reviewed articles. One was published in *Nature Epigenetics*, the other in *Soil Biology and Biochemistry*. "Both independently validated our model from Normandy," he says. "They replicated the microbial chain reactions we observed in calcium-rich burial soil, showing environmental persistence as well as epigenetic influence in plant bioassays. The echoes are real."

Ingrid narrows her eyes at the data. "Then we're on the verge of mainstream acceptance. With that also comes mainstream scrutiny. We need to get ahead of it."

"Agreed," Meera says. "No more assuming the science speaks for itself. We narrate it carefully, humbly, and with context."

As the screen flickers, there's a pause just long enough for everyone to consider what's at stake. Then Mariana smiles faintly. "Then let's move forward and document what we find. Let the data speak."

One by one, heads nod.

The next phase begins in São Paulo. A long-dormant and culturally neutral burial site on the outskirts of the city has been approved for controlled testing. Camila leads the on-site research team, with Mariana overseeing field protocols. The first experiment mirrors Meera's original design, introducing enriched microbial material to simulate a buffering zone. Its composition is carefully formulated to reflect historical micro-biomes without disrupting the surrounding ecology.

The treatment consists of dormant but viable strains of nitrogen-fixing bacteria, phosphate-solubilizing microbes, and lignin-decom-posers. All species that are commonly found in older, undisturbed wood-land soil. These strains are blended with native soil microbes from adjacent forest preserves to maintain regional compatibility. The aim is to rebalance the existing biome rather than overwrite it. As a result, they will offer a reference point for the data. Theoretically, this microbial ensemble could dilute or neutralize the residual biochemical echo left behind by long-decomposed remains. Yet equally possible, it could reawaken those fragments, catalyzing the legacy signal into sharper expression. Either outcome would be revealing.

The team expects early-stage changes in microbial diversity and nutrient cycling, shifts in carbon ratios, suppression or resurgence of opportunistic bacterial lines, and signs of microbial antagonism or inter-action. Over time, they hope to observe whether the added material accelerates decay processes, buffers microbial inheritance patterns, or alters the chemical triggers that influence epigenetic drift in surrounding lifeforms.

The team observes quietly as the biome begins to react. In the early weeks, subtle changes start to appear. Soil acidity fluctuates, bacterial expression diverges across the test zones, and nutrient profiles start to shift. Camila records each change with quiet accuracy, noting both the expected and the unexplained. The microbes, it seems, are listening. Although the message they're receiving isn't consistent.

By the second month, more persistent patterns take hold. Certain sections stabilize while others continue to drift. During the weekly review, Camila cautions the team that what they're witnessing may be only the first ripple in a much longer wave. Proper biome restructuring—shifts that endure through seasons, generations, or ecological succession—will take longer to quantify. Moreover, the epigenetic effects they're beginning to suspect, particularly those tied to developmental or reproductive cycles in plants or animals, will demand even greater patience. These are not quick-turn experiments. They are invitations to wait, listen, and let the system speak in its own time.

Five weeks into the study, the team notices distinct divergences. In one test section, the legacy signal weakens. A soft unraveling of the previously observed microbial echo. In another, unexpectedly, it strengthens. The enriched material amplifies dormant fragments, pulling legacy DNA further into expression chains. It's a split result. A paradox.

"Maybe disruption is just what resonance looks like before we understand it," Camila reflects. "The buffer either diffuses or activates the imprint, depending on the context."

Back in Hyderabad, Meera mirrors the procedure on lab-prepared plots built to mimic burial soil dynamics. Her experiments yield the same divergence. There is no pattern yet; it is just the undeniable fact that context changes outcomes. What quieted one legacy awakened another.

In Austin, Theo runs simulations based on the new data while Andrew begins mapping proximity profiles to determine what else lies near these test sites. What chemicals, minerals, or histories? They don't have answers yet.

The model has come to life, and for the first time, it's beginning to speak back.

CHAPTER 15
ECHOES BENEATH

Six months have passed since the initial soil buffering trials in São Paulo, and the world now listens with greater attention. Scientific journals began publishing early results, while media coverage, especially in directly affected regions, sparked public fascination. At the same time, peer networks strengthened and raised their voices, encouraging global institutions to take the findings seriously. The growing scientific consensus transformed a fringe curiosity into a recognized field of international inquiry. A single controlled experiment in a culturally neutral cemetery expanded into a global cohort of seven sites, each selected to represent a unique environmental and climatic profile. Together, they form a comprehensive map of how microbial buffering engages with legacy signals across diverse burial soils. The experiment now lives as a working model that is adaptable, responsive, and deeply illuminating.

The first replication took place on Vancouver Island in British Columbia. Known for its dense coniferous forests, high rainfall, and thick, acidic soil, this wet, temperate site offered a unique challenge. The region also presented an unusual pediatric trend, including small clusters of developmental delay cases that mirrored earlier findings from São Paulo and Gifu. Researchers sought to test whether the microbial buffering seen elsewhere would behave similarly in such a saturated biome. The microbial treatment here emphasized cellulose degraders and mycorrhizal fungi, organisms well suited for decomposing woody material and fostering symbiosis with forest vegetation. They expected slow response times due to the region's cool temperatures and water saturation, anticipating a sluggish microbial ramp-up and shallow integration.

The team expects gradual adaptation. Instead, within weeks, the fungal networks begin pulling the introduced microbes into their lattice, forming vast, interlaced bridges beneath the forest floor. Soil sensors light up across the grid, registering subtle shifts in carbon-to-nitrogen ratios and trace minerals on the move.

Dr. Asha Bhandari, a soil microbiologist at the University of British Columbia specializing in temperate rainforest ecosystems, leans over the monitor. "The uptake is too coordinated to be random," she says. "They're redirecting nutrient flow like it's a construction project."

Dr. Mark Ellingsen, a forest ecologist with Parks Canada who spent years studying coastal mycorrhizal webs, adjusted his glasses. "You're saying the forest just... accepted the transplant?"

"More than accepted it," Asha replies. "It's recruiting."

The data confirms it. The forest's existing fungi is dense, moisture-rich, and long established. And it has absorbed the new microbial cohort almost immediately, contradicting every model the team had built.

Dr. Mei-Lin Zhao, a biogeochemist from Simon Fraser University, stared at the projection. "We thought the density here would slow them down."

"It should have," Asha says. "In a complex network, cooperation seems to be the path of least resistance."

Rapid assimilation continues through the season. Each new reading reveals smoother exchanges, lower friction, and a steady fading of the legacy signal they had come to measure.

Mark frowns at the curve. "If the legacy's fading, what's replacing it?"

"Integration," Asha said quietly. "The past has been absorbed."

By the third month, soil cores confirmed what the graphs hinted at: reduced DNA fragment activity, lower reactive enzymes tied to legacy preservation, and a surge of lignin-degrading metabolites. These were signs that the forest absorbed the imprint and folded it into its living systems. Moisture and mycorrhizae had become its mediators, preserving the past by weaving it into a quieter, deeper register.

Yet challenges remained. Heavy rainfall caused patchy dilution in some of the control zones, leading to erratic enzyme expression and masking effects that complicated initial readings. The team proposed algorithmic dampening coefficients within the model. Adjustments that emphasized fungal dominance over bacterial variability in high-moisture environments. When updated, the model regained predictive clarity, confirming that the logic held but needed fine-grained environmental sensitivity. Vancouver Island became the wet-climate cornerstone of the system, demonstrating that saturation alters expression without erasing signal integrity.

From the temperate forests of British Columbia, the project turned its focus toward the icy latitudes of Scandinavia. The next test site was both a logistical and environmental challenge, chosen for its climate and its layered cultural significance. Unlike Vancouver, the Scandinavian site reported no unusual developmental clusters, making it a critical control for isolating environmental influence from socioeconomic or genetic factors.

The Uppsala trial began in frozen soil, literally.

Frost sheathed the tools before the first core sample reached depth, and every sensor had to be calibrated.

Dr. Linnea Sörensen, a soil ecologist from Uppsala University, crouched over a data logger wrapped in insulation foam. "Frost heave's already shifting the alignment," she said, voice muffled through her scarf. "If we don't anchor the array, it'll walk itself out of the ground before December."

Beside her, Dr. Erik Holm, a microbiologist with a reputation for patience, tapped a boot against the brittle surface. "We'll have maybe six weeks of true activity. After that, everything goes dormant."

"And then," said Dr. Freja Nyström, the youngest on the team and a mycologist who spoke of fungi like old friends, "we see who wakes up first in spring."

The three of them worked within a grid mapped carefully around the boundaries of a Lutheran cemetery. Linnea marked safe bands of soil on her tablet. "No interference with existing burials," she said. "These zones haven't been disturbed in a century. Perfect for undisturbed microbial layering."

They planted the microbial cultures in late autumn, just before the first snow, hoping to observe dormancy in real time. A slow freeze of life that would later thaw into motion.

When the spring thaw arrived, the site came alive in slow motion. Meltwater carried oxygen into the upper soil layers, and within days the sensors began recording faint metabolic pulses.

"Respiration's back," Linnea noted, scrolling through the nitrogen data. "The introduced decomposers are activating right on schedule."

Erik leaned over her shoulder. "And the psychrophiles?"

"Already moving," she said. "Native strains are reclaiming territory faster than expected."

Freja compared the live readout with the baseline. "They're not coexisting. Look at the suppression patterns. It's antagonistic."

Linnea nodded, zooming in on the molecular signatures. "Local species are degrading the foreign strains. See these reactive oxygen markers? Classic stress response."

"Could that trigger new gene expressions?" Erik asked.

"Apparently, yes." She highlighted a cluster of unrecognized sequences. "These weren't in the control group. Likely stress-induced transcriptions."

They watched in silence as irregular spikes appeared across the chemical profile. The legacy signal—the faint residue of preserved DNA they had been tracking—rose and fell unpredictably with each temperature swing.

Freja exhaled. "It's volatile," she said quietly. "Not the gentle fade we saw in Vancouver."

Linnea adjusted the sensor feed. "Here the past doesn't dissolve; it collides."

This volatility led to refinements in the growing model. Researchers suggested the integration of freeze-thaw volatility modules, adjustments that accounted for microbial dormancy, competitive surges, and abrupt phase shifts. Seasonal timing became a major factor. Predictive thresholds were extended to accommodate long delays between microbial activation and environmental triggering. The model succeeded in Uppsala by embracing volatility and demonstrating resilience in the face of chaos. Uppsala served as the control case for frozen climates, illustrating that in landscapes shaped by silence and storm, the past often returns in a rush of breath, vivid and immediate. The soil at this site responds with both sensitivity and intensity. The site served as a reservoir and functioned as a pressure valve. Through that sensitivity, the model seemed to uncover that legacy often rests in latency, yet it always holds potential energy.

Two extremes are now mapped. One is saturated and quiet, and the other is frozen and combative. The coalition turned next to a region defined by vitality, a place where microbial life never slept, and competition was fierce and adaptive. The next test would ask a different question altogether. How does the past endure through cooperation?

The site outside Arusha, Tanzania, a tropical highland site with volcanic soil and rich biodiversity, rested in quiet seclusion, ringed by acacia trees and moss-covered stones. It is hidden from the nearest village by distance and green concealment. The air is humid and sharp with the scent of wet basalt.

At the monitoring tent, Dr. Halima Njoroge adjusts a sensor stake and brushes the red dust from her sleeve. "Baseline activity's already high," she says. "These soils are alive before we even begin. Sulfur metabolizers and thermotolerant strains. This place doesn't need much encouragement."

Dr. Elias Mburu, a biochemist from the Nelson Mandela African Institution, crouches beside her, reviewing the data stream. "Then, by the model, integration should be quick. Legacy signals will dilute almost immediately."

"Should," Halima echoes.

Dr. Nia Patel, serving as the coalition's field liaison, points toward the field array. "But look here. Nutrient profiles aren't shifting. Carbon ratios and phosphorus are holding steady."

Elias frowns. "That's not possible. The introduced microbes should have disrupted the native matrix by now. Either dominance or rejection, but not this."

"It's neither," Halima says, tapping the graph. "They're coexisting. Perfect equilibrium."

They gather around the display as new readings pulse across the screen. They witness steady enzyme curves, no significant deviation in trace minerals, and a faint, unwavering legacy signal.

"It's like the system absorbed them without reacting," Nia said softly. "No spike, no fade."

Elias scans the surrounding slope where tall grasses ripple in the wind. "We expected engagement to look like conflict," he says. "Competition. But this is negotiation."

Halima smiles faintly. "Maybe this is what balance looks like in a place that's already learned to survive heat, ash, drought, and time."

Over the following weeks, the pattern holds. Nutrient levels stay within natural fluctuation ranges. Enzyme activity rises and falls with the rhythm of rainfall.

When the final assays come in, Nia summarizes the findings for the record. "The legacy signal remains unchanged. Neither amplified nor suppressed. Integration without disturbance."

Elias nods. "That's a kind of resilience we didn't account for."

Halima closes the data tablet. "Or maybe it's cooperation so deep we mistook it for indifference."

The site becomes a quiet lesson in resistance through balance. It's a reminder that in ecosystems woven this tightly, not every influence is disruptive. Sometimes, the living world simply absorbs what comes and keeps its harmony intact.

From the fertile negotiation of Arusha's microbial harmony, the coalition turned its attention to an entirely different kind of challenge. One defined by absence rather than abundance. The next site was not a biome in balance, but a crucible of extremes, where life clings to the margins and memory is etched into silence.

In the Thar Desert fringe near Gujarat, India, the challenge was dryness and temperature extremes. There's searing heat during the day, frigid nights, and rainfall so scarce it's measured in sighs. The soil here was cracked and mineral-rich, a powdery matrix of salts and silicates. Historically, this land held solitary burials, often undocumented, chosen for their remoteness. Researchers introduced a carefully selected cocktail of extremophiles, microbes capable of withstanding saline conditions, intense solar radiation, and prolonged desiccation. Expectations were modest. Early predictions leaned toward microbial death or immediate dormancy, assuming that little could persist without sustained moisture or shelter.

But the desert surprised them. Beneath the surface, within narrow fissures and shaded crevices, microclimates formed. These pockets, shielded from direct exposure and able to retain minimal traces of humidity, allowed the introduced microbial colonies to take hold. Instead of failing, they flourished. Enzyme activity picked up within days, and after two weeks, genetic assays began picking up faint yet consistent amplification of legacy DNA fragments. What intrigued the team most was the amplification. It was focused, precise, and repeatable. It seemed the harshness of the environment activated something long dormant. Legacy fragments became more chemically available, as if drawn out by adversity. Local archaeologists noted a poetic symmetry in the desert, long a symbol of silence and concealment, which now reveals its secrets. The signal here grew in coherence, and the team, marveling at the resilience of both the microbes and the memory they awakened, updated the model accordingly. The Thar Desert became a reference point for stress-induced activation, showing that environmental adversity can unmask latent genetic material. The data from Gujarat reframed hardship as a catalytic condition for biochemical expression.

From Gujarat's arid silence, the coalition shifted its focus to a region marked by complexity. An environment influenced by history, population movement, soil chemistry, and microbial diversity.

La Rioja Province, Argentina, offered the team its most volatile canvas. With its semi-arid climate and colonial graveyards, it combined historical trauma with environmental instability. The soil in this region was layered, geologically and narratively. Each stratum seemed to belong to a different era of burial practice, marked by colonial conquest, unmarked Indigenous graves, and modern agricultural overlay. Researchers adapted microbial treatments to target heavy metal leaching and phosphate regulation, two pressing issues tied to the land's previous use in mining and over-farming. Unlike other locations where the goal was to calm or buffer legacy signals, La Rioja became an experiment in exposure. From the first week, the site defied predictions.

Rather than showing a simple suppression or amplification curve, the data oscillated. The legacy signal would spike unexpectedly, fade rapidly, and then rise again without clear provocation, mirroring the sharp diurnal cycles of temperature and humidity. These swings were more than numerical; they had flavor. Chemical profiles evolved quickly, and then collapsed into silence, only to build again. Even more unsettling was the emergence of new genetic fragments. These fragments revealed evidence of deeper, previously undetected strata, distinct from any known burials. It was the only site where microbial introduction seemed to excavate the past rather than interpret it. Field archaeologists speculated that microbial agitation could be altering the bioavailability of old, mineral-bound genetic residue, pulling signals from the margins of detectability into measurable expression. In essence, the microbial treatment was revealing forgotten burials, like a sonar pulse through centuries of sediment. The team dubbed it "the echo chamber." It was the haunting rhythm of signal, silence, and revelation that repeated.

To complete the global arc of investigation, the coalition selected one final site, a region teeming with biodiversity, where legacy influence would have to compete with the chaos of living systems already at full tilt. This location would test the model's reach in the most saturated, interwoven biome yet.

Finally, Xishuangbanna, in Yunnan Province, China, presented the wettest and most biologically complex site in the study. The burial area lay within a mosaic of rainforest and farmland, surrounded by rice paddies, tea groves, and seasonal waterways. Here, the challenge was working within a system already alive with competing signals. The region's biodiversity created constant negotiation among microbes, plants, and water flow, making control difficult. To adapt, researchers blended their microbial buffer with native species, shaping it to resemble the communities found along natural forest edges. The treatments were applied gradually to avoid disruption, and sensor arrays tracked changes through the soil, plant roots, and runoff channels.

ECHOES BENEATH

The results were subtle, but profound. The legacy signal itself remained stable. Still, surrounding plant roots began exhibiting altered gene expression patterns, especially in stress-response pathways. These changes suggested that the plants were aware of the microbial shifts and were reacting to them biochemically. It was the first indication that plant systems could also register ancestral residue. Though the team handled the finding with caution, it rippled across the coalition. Legacy influence, it seemed, wasn't limited to microbial inheritance or soil-bound signatures. It was ecological. It could move across species. This prompted a major expansion to the model as it continues to evolve, allowing for cross-domain signaling and plant-microbe-gene interaction zones. What had begun as a soil study was now venturing into eco-genomics.

With the last site complete, the data floodgates opened. Teams across continents began uploading their findings into the shared archive. Threads of comparison, contradiction, and resonance wove across dashboards in Austin, Kyoto, São Paulo, and beyond. What came next was a convergence. The Xishuangbanna trial forced the research team to consider that legacy may not only echo through chemical pathways or microbial succession. It may also echo through the very organisms growing in its shadow. The soil, in this case, remembered, and it taught.

Across all six sites, the model's logic held, refined by each region's unique ecology.

The world's soils, shaped by death and time, were not uniform in their response. Some absorbed the past quietly. Others magnified it. A few whispered things no one had expected to hear. In those whispers, patterns emerged. Patterns in outcomes and in the very questions the soil seemed to pose in return.

As the data streamed back across servers and dashboards, the coalition realized they were no longer measuring change.

They were witnessing a conversation.

A global dialogue between past and present, spoken in chemistry, context, and decay.

The data from the seven global sites becomes the gravitational center of everything Andrew, Theo, and Meera do. Their meetings grow longer and more intense, moving from daily video calls to occasional in-person summits in Austin, where whiteboards bloom with molecular diagrams, soil stratification graphs, and handwritten theories on environmental resonance.

Theo builds simulation layers, translating microbial feedback loops into dynamic models that adjust based on moisture levels, mineral content, and legacy density. On a late evening in Austin, he leans back from his monitor, eyes glassy from too many hours of coding.

"It's not just a decay rate anymore," he says, half to himself, half to Meera and Andrew, who are on video. "It's a behavioral map. Each site develops its own personality, its own logic."

Andrew reviews the data, eyebrows raised. "Are you saying the soil has moods now?" He says it with just enough mock-seriousness to land like one of Theo's lines.

Theo blinks, then points at him in mock accusation. "That was my line! I knew it. You're catching the bug."

Theo pauses to reframe himself and then continues, "So, it's more like tendencies," he says while pointing to the shared screen with his mouse so they can see a visualization pulsing with slow waves of color. "Some of these systems want to absorb. Some want to echo. And others, like La Rioja, just want to mess with our heads."

Meera studies the simulation, tracing one of the branching pattern lines with her finger. "That looks like Arusha. Stable in diversity and low volatility."

"Exactly," Theo says. "It's like that ecosystem was already at peace with its history. The new microbes just folded in."

"What about Uppsala?" Andrew asks.

Theo groans. "That site's a snowstorm in a petri dish. Every time it stabilizes, the model throws off a spike. It seems to be reacting. The legacy signal there... well, it seems to flare."

Meera nods slowly. "So, what we're seeing isn't just an outcome. Its orientation. How each biome receives the past."

Theo smiles. "Bingo. That's the word I've been missing. Orientation. These are preferences more than any kind of reaction. Embedded tendencies."

Andrew folds his arms. "Then we're doing more than predicting decay curves. We're orienting the model, mapping how each site processes and expresses the genetic material."

"Which makes this," Theo says, gesturing toward his camera, "a map of styles more than a single model. A predictive framework tailored to each zone's distinct orientation."

Meera reaches for her notebook, already scribbling. "Let's not call it mood mapping, though. We'll lose every grant we've got, and Theo will start designing sticker packs for 'moody microbes.'"

Theo lights up. "Yes! You're finally thinking like me. It only took two years, but the contagion has spread!"

Andrew laughs. "If we're not careful, we're all going to catch it."

Meera brings the conversation back to the point. "Alright, alright," she says. "This is getting personal."

And it was. The more they stared at the simulations, the more the data resembled something living, temperamental, principled, and even poetic.

Andrew shifts his focus to the comparative datasets glowing across the wall-sized display. He's been tracking a trend across multiple regions. A threshold effect that continues to prove itself.

"As Meera pointed out, some of these soil types," he begins, voice measured, "they behave like capacitors. They absorb genetic signals up to a saturation point, then release them all at once like a pulse."

Meera looks up from her notes. "We're talking about a triggered response versus a steady decay curve."

Andrew nods. "Exactly. It's not linear. We're dealing with hysteresis effects. Memory with lag. The system stores the past until something like moisture, heat, or chemistry sets it off."

Theo whistles low. "The past isn't just buried. It's waiting."

"In some places, yeah," Andrew agrees. "And in others, it's leaking out slowly. Still, the capacitor model fits most of our sites. I'm running deeper comparisons tonight."

Meera, meanwhile, anchors the synthesis. She identifies common variables, flags anomalies, and stitches together the underlying principle. Context is structure.

"The model won't predict outcomes," she says, tapping the digital schematic in front of her. "It predicts tendencies and whether the soil will cradle the past or confront it."

Theo raises an eyebrow. "Are you quoting yourself now?"

"I'm quoting the model," she replies dryly. "Although, if it starts quoting us back, I want attribution rights."

Theo grins, triumphant. "That's it. You're on a roll. Our minds are now one."

Meera mock bows. "I aspire to nothing less."

Andrew chuckles, then points back to the screen. "Seriously, if the soil is reacting differently across sites, then the model's contextual. And that's what makes it predictive."

Meera nods. "Right. It's tracing a tendency in the outcome. Like a compass."

Together, they name the emerging framework the Resonance Cascade Model. It's a way of visualizing how microbial buffering either amplifies, neutralizes, or redirects legacy influence. It behaves predictably enough to build trust.

Beneath it all, something else starts to surface. A new approach and a new vocabulary. A language for talking about inheritance without chromosomes.

The Resonance Cascade Model is published to the shared international server, where every participating site is encouraged to test it, challenge it, and attempt to disprove it. What follows is three months of rigorous scrutiny. Peer labs pull apart the variables, rerun the simulations, and deploy shadow trials to expose flaws.

The model holds. In each of the six zones—wet, dry, frozen, tropical, temperate, and desert—the core predictions prove resilient. No site invalidates the model. Through the process, they reveal something more profound. Each region needs fine-tuning. The logic is solid, yet the thresholds vary.

On Vancouver Island, excess moisture muted microbial activity, extending turnover times and softening the distinction between species. Data from the rain-soaked forests showed that fungal communities dominated where bacterial variability once drove expression, prompting model adjustments to reflect high-moisture equilibrium. The site ultimately confirmed that in saturated environments, resilience arises not from speed but from balance.

In Uppsala, Sweden, freeze-thaw cycles disrupted microbial timing, creating feedback loops that produced short bursts of activity followed by long dormancy. These irregular pulses required new model parameters to capture delayed reactions and seasonal triggers. The revised approach successfully mapped microbial latency in frozen soils, showing how legacy signals reemerge only when environmental thresholds are met.

In Arusha, Tanzania, volcanic soils rich in endemic diversity resisted transformation, their microbial balance diluting outside influence. The model, built to detect sharp shifts, underestimated this cooperative stability. A new buffer index for endemic richness corrected the bias, enabling it to capture environments where legacy neither dominates nor fades but coexists in equilibrium.

In Gujarat's Thar Desert, cycles of drought and brief monsoons revealed that certain soils act like biological capacitors—storing legacy material during dormancy and releasing it when moisture or temperature shifts occur. These pulses of reactivation challenged the model's assumption of steady decay, leading to a new time-lag module that accounted for event-triggered signal releases tied to seasonal change.

In La Rioja, overlapping burial layers and past mining activity produced erratic signals that defied linear modeling. Legacy traces surged and vanished without seasonal cause, leading researchers to add a stochastic overlay to account for layered sediments and contaminants. In Xishuangbanna, China, the model stretched further when plant roots began showing altered gene expression linked to microbial shifts in the soil—evidence of cross-domain feedback where legacy influence moved beyond the microbial layer into living vegetation.

The findings expanded the Resonance Cascade Model to include plant behavior, recognizing that legacy influence moves across domains, from soil to flora to microbial networks.

With the model proven across six biomes, the coalition turned from observation to application.

CHAPTER 16
THRESHOLD

The projections begin to take shape when the coalition reconvenes for a week-long modeling sprint. Across split screens and time zones, researchers feed their datasets into a centralized system built atop Theo's resonance mapping architecture. The model is now forecasting more than it's reacting. Each simulation runs decades into the future, testing outcomes across multiple variables. Variables such as burial practices, soil buffering strategies, climate shifts, and regional chemical loads. However, three scenarios dominate the screen.

Scenario One: No Change to Current Conditions.

Scenario Two: Return to Natural Decomposition.

Scenario Three: Restoration of the Earth. Reintegrating existing entombed remains into the soil through controlled rewilding protocols and biome reactivation.

The lines across the three graphs diverge slowly at first, barely perceptible in the initial five years. Line one, representing the base-case scenario (No Change to Current Conditions), shows an increasing decline as the model rolls forward, with cumulative ecological and health impacts intensifying over time. Line two (Change-Case: Return to Natural Decomposition) arcs upward, but its momentum takes nearly two full generations to manifest clearly. By year sixty, its trajectory rises decisively above the base-case. Line three (Repair-Case: Restoration of the Earth) begins with a delayed uptick but diverges from the base-case within ten years. From there, it accelerates sharply, ultimately overtaking the change-case scenario as the most effective long-term path, illustrating that active restoration offers redemption and resilience.

Andrew leads the discussion from the shared lab with Theo. Data cascades down the screens in slow, deliberate streams. Andrew looks at the camera, making sure the coalition members can see him clearly. "Let's start with the base case," he says. "Scenario One. Baseline conditions. No change in burial practice."

Theo watches the plots unfold. "Microbial diversity drops steadily," he says. "It's a continuous decline."

"Attrition," Meera confirms. "Urban soils lose oxygen as vaults and sealed caskets accumulate. Decomposition slows, succession halts."

Julia adds from a crowded screen of faces, "The resonance metrics flatten. Activity levels approach inert conditions."

Andrew scrolls to the environmental overlays. "Groundwater nitrate profiles shift. Adjacent vegetation shows stress, reduced root density, and increased pest incidence."

Theo looks up. "And human overlays?"

"Consistent with earlier models," Andrew replies. "Small clusters of developmental anomalies grow into statistically significant bands, mostly in dense urban clusters. As this scenario rolls into decades, these regions emerge as legacy hotspots. Zones where ancestral influence is neither metabolized nor dispersed."

No one speaks for a moment. The data runs to completion.

"Scenario Two," Andrew says as he loads the next file. "The change case. Gradual transition to natural decomposition. In this scenario, legislative reforms gradually reshape burial practices. Families shift toward green burial options, incentivized by policy and driven by a growing ecological ethic."

Theo studies the curve. "The recovery's slow. Rural regions show improvement first, then suburban areas."

"Right," Meera says. "Microbial succession re-establishes in stages. Diversity indices rise at the margins before stabilizing across broader regions. Richer microbial succession returns, bringing with it the kind of active buffering that regulates legacy signals. Gradually, the resonance fields stabilize."

"Health indicators lag by two generations," Andrew observes. "But the trend is positive. Soil chemistry normalizes, agricultural yield improves."

Meera nods. "That aligns with the long-term resilience model. Restorative, but incremental. The model notes that areas adopting natural decomposition early show reduced rates of soil stagnation and more consistent recovery in surrounding flora and fauna."

"Scenario Three," Theo says. "Restoration model."

Andrew opens the final projection. "This assumes active intervention. The cessation of sealed interment and controlled reintroduction of conditioned microbial material."

Alain taps his microphone to make sure his voice comes through next on the video call. "So, the model includes disinterment and reprocessing?"

"Yes. Simulated under containment protocols," Andrew replies. "Within ten years, microbial complexity doubles in affected regions. Regions that undergo this process show dramatic biome revitalization. Genetic residue no longer accumulates; it has been recycled."

Alain appears to scan the overlay on another monitor. "Signal saturation normalizes. Nutrient lines reconnect. We see measurable improvement in soil respiration and plant vitality."

Theo exhales. "And health outcomes?"

"Positive," Andrew says. "Reduced developmental anomalies, improved baseline indicators in agricultural regions." He pauses, letting the final graphs settle on the screen. "Scenario Three yields the fastest recovery, but it's also the least practical to implement."

Meera nods. "Ethically and logistically, it's the hardest to justify."

"Still, it defines the upper boundary of what's possible," Theo offers.

Andrew acknowledges, "Scenario Three carries a high cost. This approach demands political will, financial investment, and cultural consent. In simulation, it works. In reality, it would require a global reckoning with how we relate to our dead."

Theo continues the thought. "Our view of the dead would have to transition away from viewing them as relics to be sealed away and revered. We would have to view them as a part of the continuum, still shaping the living."

The coalition sits in silence with these projections. The analytical tool they've been working on for so long has now evolved into a challenge to long-held assumptions. The model doesn't offer closure. It doesn't understand social norms and expectations. It merely offers a direction. The past, it turns out, has always been part of the forecast.

That evening, Andrew returns home to find Sonia seated at the kitchen table, laptop open beside a stack of printed research notes and a half-eaten slice of toast. The glow from the pendant light casts her face in soft shadows as she looks up. "You're late," she says, half smiling.

He shrugs off his coat and sinks into the chair across from her. "We ran the repair scenario again," he says, rubbing the bridge of his nose. "It holds. Stronger than before."

She closes her laptop gently. "And?"

He slouches slightly forward, the weight of the day still clinging to his posture. "We're facing a choice with no neutral ground," he begins slowly. "If we do nothing… If we keep sealing the dead in the ground or 'putting them on a shelf,'" he says, the last phrase clipped with frustration, "we're heading into what the team's calling a microbial winter. The soil stops breathing. The ecosystems around those sites start to decay in ways we likely can't reverse."

He pauses, watching her absorb the words. "If we change our practices now, go back to natural decomposition, the system will start to heal. It'll take time. Generations, maybe. But we'll see the trend bend upward."

He takes a breath, the next part heavier. "Conversely, if we actively reverse it and start restoring the burial grounds by pulling up what we've entombed and reintroducing them to the living soil, then we might do more than stop the damage. We might begin repairing what's downstream of it. The biological systems tied to growth, development, and cognition."

Sonia frowns. "That's still theoretical, right?"

"Of course it is," Andrew says. "We're not there yet. But the model keeps pointing in that direction. The soil's decline mirrors the same developmental irregularities we're tracking elsewhere. We just don't know how tightly they're linked."

Sonia's brow furrows. She had imagined this possibility quietly, uneasily, and in the corners of her mind. Now, hearing it spoken aloud shakes something loose. "You mean literally dig them up? All of them?" she asks, her voice softer now, more taken by the reality of what it would mean to act on something they had only ever theorized.

Andrew hesitates. "Not all at once. Not everywhere. It's staggered in the model. There are priority zones, rewilding maps, and cultural allowances. But, yes, eventually."

There's a long silence between them. The kind that only comes when the science is no longer theoretical. When it lands in the gut.

Sonia's eyes drift to the far wall, where there's an old photograph of Andrew's grandparents outside the stone steps of the Turbin family mausoleum. She pictures the roses, the hymns, the careful folding of hands during the service. Then she pictures the vault opened. The reprocessing. The return.

She swallows, the image sitting heavily in her chest. "Do you want to remove your grandparents from the family crypt?" she asks, the words careful now. "Take them out of the Turbin family mausoleum, run them through some microbial rinse, and offer them back to the earth?"

"I don't know," Andrew admits, the words dragging. "I thought I was ready for this. When it was theoretical, when it was a slide in a deck or a prediction line, I thought I could make the call. But now?"

He looks past Sonia to the window, where the trees outside sway against the dark. "Now that it's real and we're actually talking about cracking open mausoleums and releasing generations back into the ground... I just don't know how any of this scales."

Sonia nods. "It doesn't. Not yet."

Andrew adds quietly, "That's why the model's simulations start with localized restoration in limited sites. Proof of concept first."

"So, it's not about undoing everything," she offers as a statement.

"No," Andrew says. "It's about learning what can be repaired, and how far that repair extends." His voice wavers under the weight of the moment, tightened with the effort not to break. "I know I don't want to pass down a field of birth defects either. Or live in a world where the soil chokes on our sentimentality."

Sonia folds her hands together. "It's not just sentiment. It's ritual. Identity. Reverence."

He nods. "I know. That's what makes it hard. The model is clear. The science is sound. But the implications are deeply social."

They sit there, two parents, two citizens, two descendants. They no longer ask what's possible. Instead, they ask what they're willing to live with.

Sonia is the first to speak again. "If we're struggling to say this out loud to each other," she says, "what happens when we try to explain it to the public?"

Andrew exhales slowly, shoulders slumping. "They'll call it desecration. Grave-robbing. A betrayal of the dead."

"It's not," she says. "Not if we show the data. Not if we explain what's already happening. We show them what's at stake if we don't act."

He nods slowly. "We'd need to tell the story differently. Avoid charts and chemical markers. Tell the story with impact. With clarity. This is more than soil science now. It's generational ethics."

Sonia studies him. "So maybe it's time. Maybe the coalition needs to go public. Carefully. Thoughtfully. More importantly, share it openly."

Andrew doesn't respond right away. He looks down at the table, then back to her. "You think they're ready?"

"I think we'll never know until we ask."

The next morning, Sonia walks beside Andrew through the halls of Dell Children's, her steps measured, her face unreadable. The hospital buzzes with its usual energy. Apart from that energy, Sonia carries something steadier, a resolve born from the night before.

They meet Theo in the lab, where he's already scrolling through early draft visuals of the simulation outputs. He swivels around as they enter. "Well, if it isn't the brains and the conscience of the operation," he says, raising his coffee mug in greeting.

Sonia smiles faintly. "We need to talk about the public side of this."

Theo lifts an eyebrow. "The ethics release, or the PR disaster?"

"Both," Andrew says.

Sonia moves closer to the display. "We've been solely focused on risk and resolution. We need to shift. The imagery of digging up graves and reprocessing remains is going to trigger people. I don't think we lead with that."

Theo glances over. "It's not just optics. Local ordinances will shut us down before we start. Disinterment laws, zoning restrictions, and health codes. Half the regions we're modeling wouldn't even allow soil testing near burial sites."

Andrew nods. "Which is why we start with pilot zones. Controlled sites, clear regulatory pathways."

Sonia folds her arms. "The narrative is about restoration within legal boundaries."

"Exactly," Andrew says. "We'll get nowhere if this looks like policy defiance. It has to look like environmental stewardship."

"I think we frame it as legacy," Sonia says. "It's not a loss. We avoid the idea of desecration. This is continuity. Our ancestors wanted to give us a future. They saved heirlooms, passed on names, and left behind stories. They also left behind the ability to heal. To nourish what comes next. This is about accepting their final gift."

Theo stares at her for a long moment. "Damn," he says. "That's beautiful."

Andrew nods. "It reframes the narrative entirely."

Sonia continues, "We make it clear that no one's mandating this. It's an invitation. An opportunity to honor our dead with monuments and with regeneration."

Theo nods, more serious now. "Then maybe we start small. Volunteers only. See who comes forward. It gives us the chance to study public reaction and refine the rollout."

Andrew glances between them. "Pilot programs. Legacy gardens. Maybe even ritual spaces designed for remembrance and restoration."

Theo smirks. "You know, for someone who used to flinch at PR meetings, you're sounding awfully campaign-minded."

Andrew shrugs. "I'm motivated. And terrified."

Sonia smiles. "That's how you know it matters."

Before the conversation can continue, Andrew's phone begins to ring.

At the same time, Theo's computer lets out a cascade of alert chimes. All three glance at each other.

Andrew checks the screen. "It's Meera."

He picks up. "Hey, what's—"

Her voice cuts in, tight and urgent. "It's out, Andrew. The story's been leaked. Someone got their hands on the early model outputs and shared them. But they didn't include the full context. Just Scenario Three. And they're calling it—emphatically—'the recycling plan.' That word is everywhere. Headlines, hashtags, outrage. It's the only thing people are seeing."

Theo curses under his breath as he turns to the monitor, opening his inbox and coalition message threads. "It's exploding on social media. WeChat, Telegram, X, Instagram. Someone spun it as if we're launching global grave reclamation next week."

Sonia steps closer. "Who would leak it? And why only that part?"

Andrew listens as Meera continues. "We don't know who yet, but the framing is already spiraling. People think we're planning mass exhumations without consent."

Theo mutters, "Perfect. Nothing like nuance stripped from a data model to light a cultural fire."

Andrew taps the speaker button and sets the phone on the table. Meera's voice echoes in the lab, the tension unmistakable.

"We need to get in front of this," Andrew says firmly. "If we wait, the narrative solidifies. We've got to make a statement. Now."

He turns to Theo. "Get with the hospital president and the ethics committee. They need to know this wasn't us. This is not what we're proposing. We would never do it like this."

Theo nods and pushes away from the table, already reaching for his phone.

Andrew looks at Sonia, then back at the phone. "Meera, Sonia and I are going to head over to KEYE. If we can get airtime, maybe we can initiate a dialogue. Let's see if CNN or someone will pick it up for broader context."

Meera doesn't hesitate. "Do it. I'll go straight to my dean and the ethics committee. They're going to need reassurances, too. No doubt they'll demand the full model and not the cherry-picked scenario."

As Sonia drives them across town to the KEYE studio, Andrew stays on the phone, his voice low but urgent. Coalition members answer one by one, groggy in some time zones, tense in others. "We need to get ahead of this," he tells each of them. "Reach out to your benefactors, your institutional partners, and your press contacts. Calm the waters, explain what's actually happening. We need to control the narrative before it controls us."

By the time they reach the studio, Sonia has already begun drafting a unified statement in her head. "It has to be grounded," she murmurs, half to herself. "Respectful, clear, emotionally intelligent. We're not defending the science. We're inviting their understanding."

Andrew glances over. "Make it something they'll remember. Something that opens them up to the conversation that we're having."

Sonia nods, fingers moving across her tablet as she begins to write. "We tell them what this is really about. Healing. Choice. Legacy. And love. They're going to need reassurances as well. And I agree with Meera; the public will want to see the results from the full model. All three scenarios."

Two hours later, Sonia finds herself seated in the green room of the KEYE studio, the low murmur of news anchors and producers drifting in from the hallway. A young journalist not more than twenty-three, by Andrew's guess, bobs nervously between desks, balancing a clipboard and a headset.

He'd been skeptical at first, Sonia could tell. Another activist is pushing a pitch. Somehow, the social media uproar had changed everything. Now, the newsroom was hungry to fold the controversy into the midday headlines, and Sonia, well spoken, poised, and deeply informed, was their lead-in.

She had made a compelling case in the lobby, hitting the heart of the issue without inflaming it. This wasn't about exhumation or scandal, she told them. It was about truth, context, and a responsible conversation. It was about trust.

The segment producer appeared with a nod. "You're leading. One minute."

Andrew watches from just offstage, arms crossed tightly over his chest. They'd agreed it was better this way. Better optics, he had said, but also the truth. Sonia was prepared, and she was right for this moment.

He knew he came across as a scientist or a doctor. A man that is too easily painted as clinical or removed. Sonia, on the other hand, was a mother, a teacher, and someone who could speak plainly and be heard without suspicion. Her presence made the science human.

Sonia adjusts her collar and gives Andrew a glance as she's ushered to the platform. He nods once. It's all the reassurance she needs.

The lights go up, and Allison Morgan offers Sonia a practiced smile. "Mrs. Turbin, earlier today, a leaked research model ignited headlines suggesting that a global scientific coalition, a coalition you are a part of, is proposing to dig up the dead and 'recycle' them. Can you tell us, in plain terms, what's actually being proposed, and what isn't?"

Sonia doesn't look at the camera right away. She takes a breath, steadies herself, and folds her hands in her lap.

"When I was a little girl," she begins, "my grandmother used to walk me through our backyard garden. She'd pull back leaves with hands as weathered as the soil and say, 'Everything here is part of someone who came before you.' At the time, I thought she was being poetic. It was years later, after teaching biology, after becoming a mother, after walking through a hundred cemeteries for this research, that I realized she meant it literally."

She turns slightly toward the camera.

"Right now, there's a lot of fear circulating online. There are words being thrown around. Words like 'digging up' and 'recycling' miss the point entirely. So, let me offer you another word: continuity."

She pauses to let it settle.

"This isn't about desecration. It's not about robbing graves or violating memory. It's about legacy. Love. Responsibility. Our ancestors left us more than photo albums and heirlooms. They left us the Earth. And in many cases, they didn't know the ways we would shape or burden it. But we do. Now, we know."

Her voice softens and grows more resolved.

"We're part of a global coalition of researchers. Scientists, teachers, spiritual leaders, and environmental stewards. We've been studying soil health across more than a dozen countries. We've mapped microbial degradation, nutrient flow, and developmental health trends across generations. What we found is both heartbreaking and hopeful. The way we treat our dead is affecting the living."

She looks directly at the camera as though she can see the people watching.

"Every culture has understood, in its own way, that life depends on returning to the earth. Even Scripture says it—'for dust thou art, and unto dust shalt thou return.' Vaults and sealed caskets prevent that. What we're studying is a return to what nature and faith have always required."

Sonia leans in toward Allison, drawing her into the moment.

"But we also found something extraordinary. When we return to practices that allow the Earth to breathe, the soil recovers. Communities recover. Birth defect rates decline. Ecosystems strengthen. It takes time, yes. But healing is possible."

She glances briefly at Allison, then back to the viewers.

"No one is mandating anything. No one is proposing a mass disinterment. What we are doing is inviting a conversation. An opportunity. A way to honor those who came before us by letting their lives continue to give. To feed the trees, the roots, and the cycles that sustain us."

Her voice catches slightly.

"Ask yourself what your ancestors would have wanted. Would they want to be sealed away in a vault? Or would they want their legacy to be one of restoration and generosity? We believe many would choose to give back. To nourish the future. That's not recycling. That's remembering. That's purposeful."

She folds her hands again.

"We're calling for transparency, for ethics, for consent. We're calling for restoration. Restoration of the Earth, and more importantly, a restoration of trust. We're starting with this. A conversation that I'm grateful to begin with you."

CHAPTER 17
BREAKING POINT

"Damn, Andrew!" Theo exclaims, pacing with barely contained energy near his bench. "Why didn't we put her in front of the camera months ago?!"

Andrew sinks into the office chair beside him, still shaking his head in disbelief. "I know," he mutters. "She knocked it out of the park."

Theo laughs, still buzzing. "I tried, you know. Back in December, I asked her. She said she'd rather be buried alive than go on air. Guess that metaphor doesn't hit the same anymore, huh?"

Andrew chuckles despite himself. "That was... incredible. CNN picked it up within an hour. I just saw a clip. It wasn't even a full segment, just a teaser, and it already has a million views. One of the anchors called it 'an emotionally driven, respectful call to science.' And it wasn't just about the data. It was about who Sonia is. A teacher. A mother. Someone who knows how to speak to grief and hope at the same time. That clip disarmed people while also informing them."

Theo scrolls through a growing column of messages, alerts, and emails. "Sure, she gave the public the data. More than that, she gave them a story. A future. It's like she cracked open the model and let people see their families in it."

Theo continues, "I've already seen a dozen comments calling her anti-cremation. Did she actually mention it?"

"No, but the question makes sense. People think cremation's the clean alternative," Andrew responds cleanly.

Theo continues, "From an emissions standpoint maybe, but biologically it's a full stop. Once the temperature passes a few hundred degrees, there's no DNA left. There are no proteins and no viable organics. The cycle ends."

Andrew nods. "Exactly. In the model, cremation is neutral. It doesn't damage the soil, but it doesn't feed it either. No residual molecular structure means no interaction with microbial systems."

Theo frowns. "So sealed burial suspends the process, cremation deletes it, and only natural decomposition keeps the system running. That's the message we'll need to clarify. This is about continuity. Fire and concrete both close the loop, just in different ways."

Andrew agrees, saying, "Then we frame it as science rather than belief. Let the biology speak for itself. We reframe everything. Legacy, not loss. Continuity, not desecration. Now people are listening along with the experts. Families. Pastors. City councils."

Theo spins toward him, eyes brighter than they've been in weeks. "And the best part? No one's talking about the leak anymore. They're talking about gardens. Memory fields. Restorative legacy programs. Some of the threads online are surreal. People are asking how to volunteer."

Andrew nods. "It's moving fast. Too fast. But for once, it feels like it's moving in the right direction."

He glances at Theo. "Hey, how did it go with the hospital president and the ethics committee?"

Theo's expression settles slightly. "Grounded. Measured. They're leaning heavily on how the press unfolds, but no red flags yet. Looks like we still have funding, at least for now."

Andrew exhales in relief. "That's something. One less fire to put out today."

Theo gestures toward the data visualizations still hovering on the adjacent screen. "So, what's next? We got the world's attention. How do we hold it?"

Andrew's gaze narrows. "Now we show them what the future actually looks like."

Later that afternoon, the coalition gathers on a secure video call, faces lined with fatigue, hope, and cautious anticipation. For a moment, no one speaks. Then Kaoru Watanabe breaks the silence.

"So," he says, adjusting his glasses, "I assume you've all seen the broadcast?"

A round of nods and murmured acknowledgments ripple through the grid of screens.

"I've watched it multiple times," says Dr. Lotte van Dalen from Utrecht. "Each time, I feel more seen. As a researcher. As a daughter."

Meera leans into the frame from her office in Hyderabad. "We knew we needed a turning point. I just didn't expect it to come from a live television segment."

"We couldn't have scripted it better," Camila Rocha proclaims. "Now the world is watching."

"The framing worked," Dr. Nishida adds. "Framing is just the start, however. Now we need clarity."

Andrew unmutes. "That's why we're here. We have the world's attention, and now we have an obligation. Let's talk next steps."

He pauses briefly. "First, we need outside labs to pressure-test the model. Independent replication. Full transparency. If there's a flaw, it's better that we find it now. If there's strength, let it stand."

Meera nods. "I can tap two universities here in India. Maybe loop in the soil research consortium in Pune."

"I've got contacts in Wageningen and Oslo," Dr. van Dalen says. "They'll want in."

Theo chimes in next. "And someone's got to start mapping out the regulatory hurdles. If we're talking about legacy gardens, memorial restoration zones, or whatever we end up calling them, there's going to be red tape. Local zoning, environmental impact, and cultural heritage boards. We need to know what we're walking into."

"Scenario Three remains our primary model," Andrew says. "It's the only approach that shows measurable ecological recovery within a sustainable timeframe."

"I'll handle first contact with the municipalities," Camila offers. "Start with São Paulo and branch out from there."

A pause follows, then a quiet microphone tap breaks the silence. Dr. Aminata Kamara from Sierra Leone takes the primary position on the call, her face composed. "I need to speak," she says. "About the leak."

The screen grid shifts subtly as attention locks onto her.

"It came from my lab," she confesses. "I left my terminal open while stepping out for a call. One of my research assistants, a postgrad, accessed the project files and took what she thought would make headlines. She shared the most sensational interpretation of Scenario Three with the press, completely out of context."

Gasps were muffled. No one interrupts.

"She's been dismissed," Aminata continues, her voice steady despite the weight behind it. "And legal action is underway. She violated our NDA, institutional ethics, and several international policies. I take full responsibility for the lapse."

For a moment, the only sound is the gentle hiss of background noise from open mics. Then Meera offers a soft nod.

"Thank you, Aminata. That couldn't have been easy."

Meera glances around the call, her expression thoughtful but composed. "We all learned something this week. About transparency. About trust. About how fragile the story becomes when others try to tell it for us, but we move forward."

She let the words settle for a moment. "And for this coalition, by some fortune or grace, the outcome appears to be positive. The world is still listening."

Theo leans into his mic, voice encouraging. "All right, then. We've got direction, momentum, and public interest. Everyone here knows what they need to do. Start pulling threads, securing partners, and documenting everything. The chat line's open if questions come up. Keep Slack and WhatsApp running. We regroup in one week. Let's move."

That evening, in a wood-paneled fellowship hall in northern Georgia, members of the Shepherd's Stand Alliance gather for a Wednesday prayer meeting. They are a new but quickly growing branch of Christian conservatism known for emphasizing scriptural literalism, divine design, and public morality. As the group settles, a projector flickers on, and Sonia's now-viral interview begins to play.

The camera captures her composed face and steady voice. In this extended segment not aired earlier, Sonia says:

"When our daughter Junie was diagnosed with Williams syndrome, everything changed. We were told she might struggle with boundaries, might feel everything ten times more than the rest of us. But what the doctors couldn't predict, what no gene panel could define, was how her joy would transform our lives. Her presence is a daily reminder that our understanding of the human blueprint is incomplete. Not broken. Not less. Just unfinished."

She continues, voice growing stronger:

"This research doesn't erase the sacred. It honors it. Every grave holds more than a memory. It holds possibility. Every code we study carries echoes of love and loss. If you think this is about playing God, I ask you, have you ever watched a child who shouldn't have survived learn to sing? This is devotion."

The room falls silent. Then Pastor Elden Ridge stands. Broad-shouldered, silver-haired, his voice carries authority born of the pulpit. "I've read her words," he says evenly. "She's articulate, deliberate, and wrong. What they're proposing isn't stewardship; it's disturbance. They're talking about reopening graves. Digging up the dead to 'return' them, as if God's order needs correction."

His wife, Sister Marianne Ridge, folds her hands. "Scripture already tells us what becomes of us," she says. "Dust to dust. We don't need science to complete what God began. Their work treats life as a chemical cycle and disregards creation."

"If we call that renewal," Deacon Lamont Price says, "we risk forgetting where life actually comes from. They would like us to believe that it rises up from the soil. Life is a gift from God. It is given."

Elden raises his Bible. "Genesis is clear," he says. "We are formed in God's image. To suggest that life or inheritance can be restored by disturbing what He has already gathered crosses from sacred into desecration."

A murmur of assent moves through the room. The Shepherd's Stand

Alliance votes unanimously to draft a formal denunciation. Their statement will circulate by morning. A call to churches nationwide to resist what they call "the Doctrine of the Vanishing."

The document opens in solemn ritual. "We write this in sorrow and with fidelity. For though the world shifts beneath our feet and science reaches into what lies beneath, we are called to remember that the Author of Life is still present."

The Shepherd's Stand Alliance defines its stance as protection. "We support holy burial," it continues. "We oppose its undoing. The resting places of the dead are not laboratories, and the sanctity of their return to dust is not a system to be managed. The soil may hold traces of creation, but it is not the source of it. We honor the dead by leaving them in peace."

They continue, "We will accept that the child of a scientist may teach us compassion. We support their grief and the miracle, but we must not trade the certainty of sacred design for the poetry of possibility."

The final paragraphs offer both rebuke and invitation: "To every pastor, priest, rabbi, and reverent steward, we ask that you stand with us. Uphold the image of God in the face of human ambition. The Doctrine of the Vanishing is no covenant of action. It's a call to conscience. It invites us to remember what must endure, what deserves quiet coordination, and where our sacred restraint gives meaning to progress."

When the document is read aloud at Sunday services the following week, many congregants weep. Others sign their names, while a few, quietly, begin to wonder.

Three days later, Pastor Elden Ridge finds himself seated in the wood-paneled waiting room outside Senator Howard Greer's office in downtown Atlanta. The building is stately; it's a postwar federal structure retrofitted with security glass and polished marble. Yet the senator's private office, just off the corridor, tells a different story. It's one of conviction rather than politics. A large King James Bible rests open on the corner of his desk, its pages dog-eared and densely underlined. A well-worn leather chair sits behind the desk, its arms polished by decades of elbowed prayers.

When Ridge is ushered in, Greer stands to greet him with a two-handed shake.

"Pastor Ridge," the senator says, voice gravel-rich and sincere. "I read the doctrine. My staff forwarded it to me with your letter."

"I'm grateful for your time, Senator," Elden replies, settling into the seat opposite. "The doctrine is meant as a plea for spirituality and understanding. We are stewards."

Greer nods solemnly, running his fingers along the edge of the Bible.

"I'm not a biologist," he says, "but I know what it means to rest in peace. My father's buried in Covington. My mother rests beside him. If anyone disturbed that ground in the name of progress, I'd call it sacrilege."

"We're clear in what we're asking for," Ridge says. "We're asking for a moral compass. One that honors the boundary between remembrance and exploitation."

The senator folds his hands. "Then let's draw that line. I'll issue a formal call for an ethics review through the Senate Committee on Health and Human Services. We'll make the case that memory—biological or otherwise—isn't a resource to be mined."

He taps the open Bible with a gentle finality. "There are things that should remain buried, out of reverence."

Ridge nods, eyes shining. "You have our gratitude, Senator, and our prayers."

Greer offers a thin smile. "I'll take both. We're going to need them."

A quiet knock interrupts them. His aide steps in and lays a manila folder on the desk. "Sir, this just came from the state office. You'll want to see it."

Greer thanks her and waits for the door to close before opening the folder. Inside is a briefing packet, including letters from constituents and a printed medical report clipped to the front. A sticky note from his aide reads, "Local family. Donors. Urgent appeal."

He scans the first page. A child, age five, was admitted to Emory with unexplained neurological symptoms. The parents describe months of fatigue and seizures. The attached genetic workup lists a "Variant of Unknown Significance."

Greer exhales through his nose, setting the paper down slowly. "This came from my district," he says. "Just this morning."

Ridge watches him. "You see why we reached out."

Greer nods, quiet. "It's one thing to debate these matters in committee rooms. Another to see the consequences written in a family's hand-writing."

He closes the folder and rests his hand over it. "We'll look into this properly."

The senator's expression shifts to one of understanding. The line between science and sanctity, he realizes, isn't abstract anymore. It's already crossing his desk.

The next morning, Senator Greer stands before a bank of micro-phones at a press podium draped with the American flag. The seal of the U.S. Senate gleams beneath the studio lights as reporters jostle for position.

"In the name of moral clarity and human dignity," Greer begins, "I am formally requesting a bipartisan ethics review into current soil-based genetic recovery research. We must ensure our pursuit of knowledge does not violate the sanctity of the grave. Scientific advancement must never come at the expense of spiritual peace."

He speaks without notes, quoting Scripture and invoking the Founding Fathers in equal measure. "We are more than bodies and data. We are memory and meaning. Our dead deserve solemn care."

Within hours, the story trends nationally. Conservative media plat-forms herald Greer's call as a courageous stand for values. The headline on one major outlet reads, "Faith vs. Futurism: Senator Calls for Line in the Sand."

Cable news splits in coverage. On one network, a panel praises the move as long overdue, a necessary moral boundary in an age of unchecked innovation. Another features a tense debate between leading geneticists defending the research as essential to understanding genetic inheritance, and parents of children with rare disorders who plead for continued discovery.

Social media ignites. #DoctrineOfTheVanishing gains traction along-side #LetThemRest and #SacredSoil. Celebrities post filtered images of cemeteries with the caption "Not your lab."

Meanwhile, in university labs and think tanks around the world, scientists begin preparing for scrutiny. Among them, a few pause out of respect more than guilt. Whether they agree or not, they understand the story has changed. The language of legacy now has an echo in scripture.

For the first time since Sonia's broadcast, the public has grown silent on what can be done and is now asking what should be done.

Later that evening, the coalition regathers on a secure video call. Four squares light up the screen. Andrew in a dimly lit office, Theo with a cup of something steaming, Meera seated before a bookshelf of scientific journals, and Sonia quiet and composed at the kitchen table.

"Do we respond?" Andrew asks, breaking the silence. "Publicly, I mean. We've lost a week of narrative. Greer's speech is everywhere."

"We're losing ground," Theo adds. "People remember feelings more than the data. Sonia, they listened to you. We need that again."

Sonia shakes her head. "No. Getting back in front of a camera makes this a debate. It's not about who speaks louder or who cries harder on national television."

She pauses, voice steady and resolute. "This is about science. It's about human life; future human life. If we turn this into a contest of rhetoric, we lose the very thing we're trying to protect." She leans closer to the screen. "The second we start debating in public, we shift the burden from truth to persuasion. We reduce it all to opinion, and opinion isn't what brings someone back from the edge of a diagnosis. Data does. Treatment does. Time and trust and repeated results."

She looks briefly off-screen, then back. "Greer wants this to be a cultural battleground, but we are stewards, and stewardship means doing the quiet work, even when it's unpopular."

Just then, Junie wanders into the kitchen, asking for help reaching a book from the shelf. She looks into the camera, having heard the debate while she approached. "God was the first scientist," she says, as if it's the most obvious thing in the world. "He made water and air and clouds and rain. He even made dirt smart."

Sonia presses a kiss to her daughter's temple, and for a brief moment, the call is quiet. Each of them is struck by the simple truth in a child's voice.

Sonia follows Junie back out into the living room to retrieve her book.

Meera nods, slowly, still looking at the space Junie left behind. "She's not wrong, you know. That might've been the most coherent theology of science I've heard all week."

She shifts her gaze back to the screen, more grounded. "So, what's next?"

"We document," Theo says. "We verify. We publish. Then we let the work speak for itself."

Andrew sighs. "We better make sure that work is unassailable."

Within days, an emergency session of the U.S. Senate Subcommittee on Science, Ethics, and Public Trust is convened. The hearing chamber on Capitol Hill hums with press, aides, and staffers, the air dense with anticipation and the faint scent of old paper and polished wood. Dark blue carpets stretch beneath high-arched windows, and the committee seal hangs prominently behind the panel bench. This is where spectacle and scrutiny converge.

A leather-bound Bible sits prominently on the dais before the chair, bookmarked with ribbons and visibly worn at the spine. The presence of faith in the chamber is unspoken, yet palpable.

Meera and Andrew are invited to testify. Though remote testimony is permitted, Meera flies in from Hyderabad, driven by a conviction that her presence must be felt in the room. She wants them to see her and not just her data. Dressed plainly, she and Andrew stand side by side beneath the council seal, speaking as scientists trying to illuminate rather than persuade.

Meera opens with the context of genetic drift, historical silence, and the quiet revelations in soil. Andrew follows with the implications for neurodivergence, inherited trauma, and species resilience.

Some senators listen with reverent attention. A representative from Vermont praises their courage and clarity. A junior senator from Oregon expresses admiration for their measured tone and scientific integrity, but not all voices are aligned.

Senator Melton from Mississippi warns of cultural desecration, invoking the traditions of Southern burial grounds and generational memory. Senator Alvarez from Texas calls for an immediate halt to any federally funded exhumation initiatives, citing concerns over community unrest and religious infringement. Senator Roman of New Jersey proposes a moratorium until a bipartisan ethics panel can conduct a full review of the implications for both public health and cultural respect.

Then, a stern and sharp voice from the back asks whether the coalition will proceed without universal consent.

Meera's answer is simple. "No. Science without consent is not progress. It's colonialism."

That line lands like a bell. Some murmur in agreement. Others shift uncomfortably in their seats.

The Senate recesses with no consensus, but one truth is clear. The world is no longer indifferent.

CHAPTER 18
SACRED GROUND

The Senate Subcommittee on Science, Ethics, and Public Trust reconvenes after lunch, this time behind closed doors. The public hearing earlier that day ignited more questions than consensus, and the morning's display of passionate testimony, emotional appeals, and media flashbulbs left many senators rattled. Some moments were too raw, too personal for soundbites. Others are too speculative to stake a claim in front of a national audience. And so, in this second session, the cameras are shut off, the gallery emptied, and the press held at bay.

Without the glare of the spotlight, the atmosphere shifts. What was once posturing becomes process. Senators who had delivered fiery monologues hours earlier now speak in moderated tones, asking real questions rather than rhetorical ones. The room is smaller, quieter, and designed for deliberation rather than declaration. They return with fewer staffers and lowered voices, the morning's testimonies still echoing faintly in the corridors outside.

The focus now is ethics. They discuss what the coalition has discovered and how science should move forward in a world still tethered to faith and fear. Experts from the National Institutes of Health (NIH), academic institutions, and bioethics centers take the floor in rotation, grounding the conversation in decades of precedence and cautionary tales. Representatives from NIH, the federal agency leading biomedical and public health research in the United States, offer a particularly grounded perspective. Their testimony draws on decades of experience balancing scientific advancement with patient protections, informed consent, and public trust. They recall lessons from landmark projects like the Human Genome Project and the evolution of federal standards around genetic privacy, emphasizing that progress must walk in step with prudence.

A professor of medical ethics from Johns Hopkins begins her remarks with the challenge, "Science can move faster than ethics. When it does, however, we must ask, what are we moving faster toward? And for whom?"

The committee listens as testimony unpacks the frameworks of informed consent, ancestral rights, and the emerging concept of "resting sovereignty." It's the idea that the dead, though silent, still possess a form of moral agency. Several senators exchange glances, aware that cemeteries have been moved for highways, developments, and even shopping centers. The precedent isn't new. What's different now, the witnesses argue, is intent. These studies don't relocate the dead for space or convenience, but for access to whatever still lives within them. Some senators scribble notes. Others stare straight ahead, visibly torn.

Andrew is present for the hearing and submits written testimony in addition to appearing in person. His contribution outlines the data collection protocols, the coalition's internal review procedures, and the ethical framework they've adopted to ensure respect for all human remains involved in the study. Though his voice is not heard aloud in the session, the pages he submits serve as a technical counterbalance to Meera's moral and philosophical appeal.

Meera speaks again, briefly this time. Her voice is calm and unwavering.

"This isn't just a scientific pivot," she tells them. "It's a moment of reckoning. If our pursuit of knowledge cannot coexist with dignity, then we've misunderstood the purpose of knowledge altogether." She pauses, then continues, "Medical history is filled with moments where we took leaps of faith, where the science wasn't perfect, but the stakes demanded courage. We transfused blood before we understood all its types. We administered anesthesia before we mapped the brain. We decoded the genome before we knew what most of it meant. These weren't acts of recklessness. They were acts of respect for life, for suffering, and for the possibility of healing. This is one of those moments. The unknown doesn't exempt us from responsibility. It invites us to meet it with both humility and hope."

By day's end, the session closes without resolution. Even without answers, the tone has shifted. What began as a political skirmish is now evolving into something quieter, deeper. It's a national reflection on what science can do and what it ought to become.

That evening, just after 9 p.m. in London, the coalition regroups on a video call. Theo, Meera, Andrew, Sonia, and half a dozen international partners appear in little squares across time zones. No one speaks for the first few moments.

Theo finally breaks the silence. "So, that was a soft *maybe* from Washington. About as firm as pudding."

Andrew sighs. "It's better than a no, and they didn't accuse us of heresy this time."

Sonia gives a wan smile but says nothing.

Then the news comes in. A university hospital in southern Europe, one of the coalition's earliest and most active partners, has received conditional approval from its national health board to proceed with a controlled exhumation study. The site in question lies on the outskirts of a rural municipality, a modest cemetery whose records stretch back centuries.

The graves selected are over a hundred years old. Some date back to a local cholera outbreak; others were marked simply as "Unknown." Before approval was granted, the research team spent weeks combing regional archives, church registries, and municipal birth and death records, seeking any living descendants or recorded ties. No claims surfaced. Notices were posted in the local paper, and a public hearing was held with only a handful of attendees, none of whom opposed the motion.

The site was chosen precisely for its anonymity and for its apparent detachment from any living familial legacy. The hospital believed it had found the one place where science might quietly proceed, respectfully, methodically, and without controversy.

The coalition receives the news with cautious optimism. It is the first concrete opportunity to test their methods under tightly controlled ethical oversight. They agree to move forward, eyes open and breath held.

The team holds its collective breath.

Within twenty-four hours, the local newspaper runs a front-page headline about the study, branding it "Scientists to Unearth Forgotten Dead." The article, though factually accurate, is framed in a way that stirs unease. Words like "dig," "probe," and "reclaim" ripple through the community, igniting dormant tensions.

By morning, protesters gather at the cemetery gates. Some carry handmade signs; others wear mourning black. A few kneel on the ground in silent prayer. Though peaceful at first, the crowd grows by the hour, stoked by regional influencers and inflammatory social media posts.

By late afternoon, a confrontation erupts. Misinformation spreads quickly that the scientists are disturbing recent graves, and that children's remains are among those being studied. Riot police are called in. Gravestones are toppled; some are shattered beyond repair.

In the chaos, someone hurls a heavy stone through the back window of the equipment van, narrowly missing a technician crouched inside. Several protesters breached the perimeter fence, their shouts mixing with the static of police radios. In the scuffle, a field researcher is struck by a length of broken signage, thrown blindly from the crowd. He collapses just steps from the cemetery gate, clutching his arm.

Later, an X-ray reveals a clean break to the radius, along with torn ligaments and heavy bruising to his shoulder and ribs. The study is immediately suspended. Police escort the team to a temporary safehouse while the site is placed under lockdown.

What was meant to be the coalition's most cautious, ethically sound step forward instead becomes a flashpoint. One that none of them saw coming so swiftly or so violently.

Theo stares at the screen, stunned. "They were nameless. Completely unclaimed."

Meera shakes her head. "Not to the people who live there. Not to the ones who buried someone else nearby. Grief radiates outward; it's not a closed system."

Sonia whispers, almost to herself, "So does fear."

Elsewhere on the new political and emotional landscape, Senator Greer sits quietly in the guest room of his daughter's house, the day's headlines folded on the edge of a borrowed desk. The furnishings are modest with family photos on the walls, a hand-drawn family portrait taped to the door, and children's books stacked in neat piles. His wife, Margaret, stands behind him with a mug of chamomile tea, her free hand resting gently on his shoulder.

They had come down for a long weekend after their granddaughter, Anna, had a brief illness, just a fever that lasted longer than expected. Their daughter had seemed relieved to have them close. It was more than logistics; it was instinct. Greer, who once found refuge in the routines of the Senate, now found himself grounded by the smaller, steadier rhythms of family life.

Anna is the kind of child who draws suns in every corner of the page and narrates her thoughts while tying her shoes. She's a question factory. That week, her second-grade class had started a "Family Roots" project, mapping where everyone came from. She'd asked her grandfather if bones could tell stories the way books do. The question, innocent and impossible, had lodged somewhere deep.

It isn't the fever that unsettles them. It's the echo of her curiosity, arriving at a time when Greer's professional life is consumed by talk of the body, burial, and the unseen life of memory in the soil. For the first time, the hearings and headlines feel close enough to touch.

Margaret watches her husband carefully, sensing that proximity. "You keep rereading that transcript," she says softly. "The one from Dr. Rao?"

He nods without looking up. "She's thoughtful. Careful with her words. I don't know yet if I agree, but she believes what she's saying."

"She reminds me of someone," Margaret says, setting the tea beside him. "Someone who's still trying to believe in both faith and reason."

He smiles faintly. "You always did have a way of finding the middle."

"I'm just tired of people choosing sides," she says. "When Anna asks where we come from, she isn't asking for a theory. She's asking to belong."

The room falls quiet, the television murmuring in the background. Coverage of the hearings is replayed on a twenty-four-hour loop. On screen, Dr. Rao's measured cadence fills the room. Her tone is firm while remaining compassionate, describing knowledge as a covenant.

Margaret moves closer, her voice almost a whisper. "I read about the woman who spoke after the protests—Sonia, wasn't it? Her daughter has Williams syndrome. She said something I can't stop thinking about. That remembrance and research aren't enemies, just two ways of loving what came before."

Greer looks at her, surprised by the reference.

"I don't know if we can trust all this science," she says, "but I know what it feels like to love a child you can't explain. And I know what it means when someone stands up and says that love still matters."

Greer doesn't reply. He only turns back to the screen, the senator's certainty beginning to yield to something quieter and more human.

That evening, while the house settles into its soft suburban silence, Margaret remains awake beside the phone. She rereads an article that quoted Sonia's advocacy work. The words feel humble and unfinished, full of the same uncertainty that now colors her own faith.

With hesitant courage, she looks up Sonia's public educator profile and dials the number.

Sonia answers on the second ring, her voice cautious. Margaret introduces herself. The call begins haltingly, two women divided by belief but united by something elemental: the ache of loving without needing complete understanding.

They talk about the children, the gaps between science and scripture, and the courage to live without neat answers. Sonia describes Junie—her daughter's music lessons, her joy, her unfiltered way of being. "She doesn't wait for the world to make sense," Sonia says. "She sings anyway."

Margaret smiles through the ache. "Anna sings too," she says. "Mostly when she thinks no one's listening."

"Then they'd get along," Sonia replies.

For a long while, they say very little. The silence between them feels sacred. It's a space where empathy can breathe without trying to persuade.

Margaret discusses her daughter Caroline's worry about the sermon she's rewriting in light of the hearings. "She wants to believe the world is still guided by grace," she says. "But grace feels smaller lately."

"Maybe grace isn't smaller," Sonia offers gently. "Maybe it's just closer than we thought."

When the call ends, Margaret rests in the stillness, hand still on the receiver. She looks toward the hallway where a faint nightlight glows outside Anna's room. Something inside her, the way she carries her convictions, has shifted.

The next morning, she tells Caroline about the call. They stand in the kitchen as the kettle whistles itself hoarse on the stove. "I didn't call to argue," Margaret admits. "I called because I needed hope, and I found someone who hasn't given up on it."

Caroline says nothing at first. Then she reaches across the counter and takes her mother's hand. "Then maybe that's what we bring, hope."

Two days later, they stand together on the steps outside the Senate building, outside the same building where the ethics subcommittee had convened. The morning light is thin and cool; the plaza below is dotted with reporters setting up tripods and cables. Margaret had called the local press herself, quietly leveraging her position as the wife of a sitting senator to make sure cameras are rolling when they arrive.

She didn't do it for spectacle. She did it because the conversation drifted too far from the people it is meant to protect. Every headline now carries the language of policy and conflict, but none speak of families. Of the parents who lie awake at night reading medical journals they barely understand. Of children who ask impossible questions about life and belonging.

Margaret believes that if the public can see faces and hear the voices of a mother instead of a senator, they might remember why the debate matters at all.

Caroline hesitates at first. "What if it looks political?" she asks.

"It will," Margaret confirms. "But sometimes politics needs a reminder that it's about people. If we stay silent, they'll fill the silence for us."

So they're here—mother and daughter, faith and doubt side by side—to offer something the headlines leave out. A voice for the families caught in the space between science and solace. A reminder that progress, without compassion, risks forgetting who it's meant to serve.

Now, as the air turns crisp around them, the crowd gathers in a loose half circle. Reporters stand poised, microphones angled forward, their red lights blinking.

Margaret steps to the podium first, her voice steady. "We're not scientists," she begins. "We're not here to argue data or doctrine. We're here because families are watching. Because our children and grandchildren will inherit whatever we decide in rooms like this."

She steps back, and Caroline—nervous and resolute—takes the microphone. A pastor by calling, she never imagined herself addressing cameras. But when she thinks of Anna's drawings and endless questions, her fear loosens its hold.

"My daughter once asked why the moon follows our car at night," she says, a small smile flickering. "I told her it's because light finds a way to stay with us. Science doesn't have to erase faith. Curiosity doesn't erase compassion. We're not asking you to take sides. We're asking you to remember who lives on the other side of your decisions."

Margaret returns to the podium to close. "Before you write laws or headlines, before you draw your lines," she says softly, "think of the children who will live inside those lines. Ask yourself not what is popular, but what is human."

For a moment, the microphones catch nothing but silence. The collective stillness that comes when conviction meets empathy. Somewhere in the crowd, someone exhales shakily, the sound barely audible but unmistakably human.

CHAPTER 19
BENEATH AND BETWEEN

One month has passed.

The media frenzy has finally begun to recede, its appetite dulled by newer controversies and fading novelty. While the story of genetic absence and buried memory still surfaces in academic journals and the occasional long-form editorial, the headline chaos has softened. In its place, something quieter has emerged, space to work.

The Senate ethics committee, after extended deliberation, has authorized continued development and testing of the predictive model, albeit under heightened oversight and strict site-by-site protocols. Notably, Senator Greer abstained from the vote, citing an apparent conflict of interest due to prior involvement in one of the early international symposiums that informed the coalition's research trajectory. For the coalition, this marks the first real opportunity to operate beyond theory. The fieldwork can now begin in earnest.

The approval, however, came with unexpected support from an unlikely corner — though not because that corner had changed its stance. Weeks earlier, a growing evangelical group, the Shepherd's Stand Alliance, had published a widely circulated statement known as the Doctrine of the Vanishing. It condemned the coalition's work, framing burial as a sacred act of remembrance and warning against any attempt to "resurrect the flesh for the purpose of rewriting creation." Yet the document's opening line, "We honor the dead by burying them," was swiftly lifted from its context and adopted by supporters of the science as a moral defense. If burial was indeed an act of honor, they argued, then understanding what the earth now held was an extension of that same integrity. The coalition's mission, once framed as desecration, was reframed as devotion. Scientists were not unearthing the past to disturb it. They were honoring the dead in the most literal sense by paying attention to what remained.

With the ethics committee's decision in hand and public sentiment shifting ever so slightly in their favor, the coalition turns its attention to logistics. The team's first full-scale, fully sanctioned exhumation is scheduled to take place on Hart Island, just off the coast of the Bronx in New York City. This decision followed weeks of discussion within the coalition as they reviewed five possible sites around the world. Each with its own haunting logic.

In Italy, Poveglia Island offered a historical weight that few places could match. Once a quarantine station during plague outbreaks, the island was layered with mass burials and sealed tombs dating back to the eighteenth century. Yet its very history made it unsuitable. Centuries of epidemic response had sealed the ground beneath vaults meant to isolate disease from soil and water. Disturbing that equilibrium risked both contamination and outrage. Even with its layered potential, the site remained off-limits. It's a haunting reminder of how burial itself evolved to keep the living safe from the dead.

Germany's Beelitz-Heilstätten, a crumbling sanatorium complex outside Berlin, presented another option. Adjacent wartime burial sites held unclaimed remains, likely sealed and layered with the trauma of two world wars. Yet concerns over historical sensitivity and potential military entanglements gave the team pause.

On the other side of the globe, Pulau Galang in Indonesia once served as a refugee camp for Vietnamese boat people. There, dozens of unmarked and sealed graves lingered on overgrown land, untouched since the 1980s. But political complications and environmental volatility in the region made approval uncertain.

In Brazil, the coalition considered Vila Formosa in São Paulo. It's one of the largest cemeteries in Latin America, which received a surge in rapid, sealed burials during the height of the COVID-19 pandemic. It offered scale, anonymity, and recency. The qualities are valuable for comparative study. Though early discussion raised concern about residual infection, the science was clear: viral material cannot survive the chemistry of death. The hazard was never biological but cultural, tied to grief too recent and memories still raw. What the site lacked, however, was the layered chronology needed to study generational progression.

Ultimately, Hart Island offered something none of the others could. It offered a structured chronological layout. For over 150 years, the island has served as New York City's potter's field, a place of rest for more than a million unclaimed or indigent dead. Bodies were buried in simple pine boxes, stacked in long trenches, often sealed by pressure and time. Burial locations shifted roughly every decade, offering a built-in linear map of time, ideal for tracking genetic change or erosion across generations.

Some of those buried were victims of epidemics or economic despair. Others had simply fallen through the cracks. Their names may be lost, but their remains still carry the imprint of when they lived, and perhaps, what changed as they died.

Importantly for the coalition's research, Hart Island's burial practices follow a temporal grid. Each trench is a silent archive of its time, organized chronologically rather than by name or heritage. The team believes this unique structure offers an almost ideal testing ground for their model, enabling a stepwise examination of genetic patterns over time. Their theory is that genetic memory or degradation manifests incrementally across generations. If that theory is correct, then Hart Island could make those subtle shifts visible with chilling clarity.

Preparations are already underway. Meera, Andrew, and Theo will be on-site with a small contingent of field researchers. City officials have issued the necessary permits, and collaboration agreements are in place with the Department of Corrections and NYC Public Health. A mobile lab will be stationed nearby, along with temporary field housing for sample containment, live data streaming, and immediate analysis.

The island, long closed to the public, has rarely known such scrutiny.

Still, for the coalition, it is sacred ground. It's valuable not simply for who lies beneath, but for what those remains might still teach the living.

At the next collaborative meeting, attention turns to personnel. The coalition agrees that the emotional weight of fieldwork can't be ignored. Memories of Normandy and of the silence, the resistance, and the unshakable grief still hang over those who were present months earlier. The leadership team makes it clear that anyone who participated in the Normandy visit was permitted to sit this one out. Hart Island would be more immersive, more immediate.

Still, hands go up.

"I'll go," says Julia van Eyk from Utrecht, her voice calm but steady. "I was in Normandy. I remember every moment of it, but I also remember what it meant. I feel a responsibility to be there."

No one challenges her. A few nod. Her presence anchors the effort, a reminder that empathy and resolve can coexist. Alain Fournier, the French forensic specialist who helped lead the team in Normandy, is next to speak.

"I'll go too," he says. "Normandy was difficult and more than I expected. But I want to see this through. We've come too far to look away now."

Others follow, balancing scientific eagerness with quiet apprehension. Each name added to the roster carries its own logic. Volunteers bring experience in pathology, fluency with on-site protocols, and emotional resilience.

The list fills up fast. Fourteen scientists in total signed on within the hour, each supported and funded by their hospitals and universities. This isn't an expedition of detached observers. It's a reckoning, and a truly global one.

Within a week, all fourteen scientists arrive in New York. Most check in at the Residence Inn by Marriott near the Bronx Terminal Market. It's an unassuming hotel with long-stay amenities, and it's within walking distance to the ferry terminal at City Island that grants restricted access to Hart Island. It's as close as city infrastructure allows. The rooms are modest but clean, and the staff, having been briefed in advance, treat the guests with a blend of curiosity and respect.

From the upper floors, some rooms offer a faint view of the East River and the hazy outline of the island itself. At night, the city hum remains distant, softened by the hotel's insulation and the weight of the task ahead. Laptops glow late into the evening. Hallway conversations turn quiet and clipped. Everyone knows why they're here and what's about to begin.

On the fourth floor, three doors in a row bear familiar names. Julia, Alain, and Theo have been assigned adjacent rooms. It's an arrangement that feels deliberate, a quiet acknowledgment of what they shared in Normandy.

Theo knocks lightly on Julia's door, then leans against the hallway wall, coffee in hand. He speaks loudly, "If I start sleep-talking about bone erosion and methylation drift, someone please intervene. Preferably with coffee. Or a bagel."

Julia opens the door, already smiling. "No promises on the bagel, but I'll record it for the archives. Might be your most coherent theory yet."

Alain steps out of his room just as Theo delivers an exaggerated bow. "The oracle of Utrecht speaks."

"You're both ridiculous," Alain says, but there's a glint of relief in his eyes. "Still, I'm glad it's us here. Familiar faces. Familiar ghosts."

Theo raises his cup. "To ghosts, then. And to not letting them win."

Julia nods. "And to remembering why we came."

For a moment, no one speaks. The hallway hums with silence and distant elevator chimes.

Then Julia glances down the hallway and places herself a little closer to the others. "I never thought I'd be *here* again," she says quietly. "My father was a gravedigger. Old school, with wooden shovels and careful hands. When I was little, I didn't understand any of it. Cemeteries just felt heavy and strange, but as I got older, I realized he saw them differently. To him, they were libraries with secrets buried in dirt. I think that's why I stayed in this work, even after everything."

Alain looks over, his brow raised. "That explains a lot," he says warmly and with a touch of sarcasm, "I used to be a field artist before I went into forensics. Sketching remains, structures, and crime scenes. At first, it felt investigative. Then it started to feel like witnessing. Like giving shape to something no one else would look at."

Theo whistles, mock-impressed. "Here I thought I was interesting because I own a lava lamp and once solved a Rubik's Cube in the dark. You two are carrying entire novels."

They laugh. A genuine, short, and needed laugh.

Then, almost in unison, they retreat back into their rooms, but not before Theo pulls a small bottle of Scotch from his bag and raises an eyebrow. "One sip. For science. And solidarity."

Alain smirks and nods. Julia hesitates, then shrugs. "Just a sip."

They share the drink quietly in the hallway, passing the bottle between them like a ritual. No toasts, no speeches. Just presence.

When they finally part ways, there's a gravity to the silence that follows. They each move past the weariness and carry a personal connection; a sliver of light held between them like a shared breath.

The next morning, under a muted sky, the team boards a chartered ferry authorized for research access to Hart Island. The public hasn't been permitted here for years, and the privilege of entry lends the air a certain gravity. The crossing is quiet, save for the rumble of the engine and the occasional gull. As the island comes into view, the mood sharpens. Anticipation is left unspoken. Everyone knows their roles.

Upon arrival, they find the terrain is wind-beaten, overgrown in places, and dotted with remnants of buildings long since abandoned. The island's silence feels heavier up close, broken only by the crunch of gravel and the low murmur of logistical briefings.

Representatives from the Department of Sanitation, the Department of Corrections, NYC Public Health, and the Parks Department are already on-site, clustered near the portable field lab and supply tent. The Parks Department, which officially took ownership of the island in 2019, brings historical context and custodial oversight to the operation. Each representative has a clipboard and a cautious expression. They are here to oversee and not interfere, but their presence is unmistakable. The ferry that brought the coalition remains docked nearby, repurposed as a commissary and restroom hub. With no public infrastructure on the island, it becomes a shared lifeline. Its galley is stocked with boxed lunches and thermoses of coffee, its lower deck offering the only working toilets within reach. The boat hums quietly in the background, a link to the mainland and a reminder of the island's isolation.

The coalition begins its work by establishing soil research stations across pre-approved zones. These are clear areas away from known burial trenches. Each station is GPS-mapped, gridded, and flagged, then logged into the live monitoring system. Initial readings include pH, salinity, temperature, moisture content, and microbial presence. The deeper work, however, lies in the analysis of viability and genetic composition.

Soil cores are extracted using sterile borers and sealed immediately in numbered, tamper-proof containers. The mobile lab, assembled aboard the ferry and equipped with portable centrifuges and nanopore sequencers, enables immediate baseline testing before samples are transferred to a complete laboratory facility. On-site, the researchers measure DNA trace density, looking for nucleic acid fragments that may have migrated into the soil over time. They quantify the integrity of those fragments by measuring how much has degraded, how much remains viable, and whether any signatures suggest lateral genetic drift.

They also scan for specific sequences that may signal the presence or absence of expected biological markers across decades. This includes human genetic material as well as plant, fungal, and bacterial DNA. The decomposition process and the soil environment potentially impact each. Isotope ratios are tested to determine the soil's chemical history, including possible contamination or changes in elemental composition. Every sample becomes a layered record of time, interaction, and erasure.

Every container they seal carries weight, not just in its potential data, but in its proximity to the sacred and the unknown.

By the end of the first day, the rhythm has set in. Extraction, labeling, data entry, and documentation. The team rotates through soil stations with quiet focus, recording everything with methodical precision. Small adjustments are made as patterns begin to emerge. Some samples are richer than expected, others offer only silence. The sun breaks through only once, casting long shadows across the field station tents and worn footpaths. From a distance, it looks almost like an archaeological survey, but the urgency and the reverence make it something else entirely.

The team returns to the hotel that evening as the sun drops behind the silhouetted warehouses and smokestacks along the East River. Andrew finds Meera seated near the back of the lobby, notebook open, fingers tapping quietly on its spine.

"Mind if I join you?" he asks, sliding into the chair beside her.

She glances up, offers a tired but genuine smile. "Please. I was hoping to debrief while it's still fresh."

Andrew sets a tablet on the table between them. "We logged seventy-four samples today. Good distribution across the northern grid. We already flagged five for early sequencing. One of them has elevated nucleotide concentrations, well above baseline."

Meera leans forward, alert. "Already? From surface layer cores? That's fast."

"Faster than we anticipated," Andrew says. "Theo thinks it might be due to hydrological drift from a denser trench nearby. We'll need a deeper core to verify. But if it holds…"

Meera nods, finishing the sentence in her head. "Then we might have a measurable gradient."

They sit in quiet agreement for a moment. Then Meera says, "I saw Alain pause during one of the collections. He looked slightly over-whelmed and reverent. I think he recognized something in the soil."

Andrew folds his hands. "Everyone did, in their own way. Even the Parks rep got quiet when we flagged the perimeter. Like we were mapping something sacred."

She closes the notebook. "We are."

He smiles. "Then day one goes in the book as a success. Not just for the model, but for the people doing the work."

Meera lifts her tea. "To tomorrow, then."

Andrew raises an invisible glass. "To the living, and to those still speaking."

Day Two begins before the sun clears the low haze over the East River. Julia and Alain, already suited up and reviewing the day's assignments, catch sight of the posted rotation chart near the ferry ramp.

"We're split," Julia murmurs, scanning the team breakdown. "Different sample zones."

Alain looks over her shoulder, frowns. "Can we swap?"

Theo, overhearing as he steps onto the dock with a breakfast bar in hand, raises an eyebrow. "Trouble in paradise?"

Julia half-smiles. "We work better together. And we're both comfortable near the trench edges. That should count for something."

"It does," Alain adds. "We don't rush. We don't flinch."

Theo takes a bite of his breakfast and shrugs. "I'll flag it to Meera. She's been open to rotation tweaks."

By the time the team sets foot back on Hart Island, Julia and Alain are walking together, kit bags slung over their shoulders, boots crunching against dew-wet gravel. Their assigned grid hugs the southern perimeter of the 1980s burial trench. It's a site heavy with volume, even if it hasn't been analyzed yet.

They work in sync, neither needing to speak much. Occasionally, they pause out of ceremony more than for rest. Even through gloves and masks, they feel the gravity beneath their feet.

Julia kneels near a flagged post and brushes aside a leaf. "The layout still gets to me," she says quietly. "You can feel the decade, somehow."

Alain nods without looking up. "It's the silence. That's what I felt in Normandy too."

A breeze moves across the open field, lifting fine grit into the air. They pause together, standing at the edge of something unseen, but deeply known.

By day five, the soil phase is complete. Every scheduled grid has been sampled, cataloged, and sealed for sequencing. The field stations have been packed down, and most of the mobile lab work has shifted back to Manhattan for longer-term analysis. Now, the focus turns to what comes next, the exhumations.

It begins with quiet protocol checks and sterilization procedures. A small contingent from the city's Office of Chief Medical Examiner observes each step, documenting compliance with excavation standards. The team will proceed one generation at a time, starting with the earliest tract designated by burial decade. The 1940s trench, buried furthest from the ferry dock and closest to the tree-lined boundary at the island's northeast end, has been cleared for excavation.

The atmosphere shifts. Field science gives way to something more intimate, an encounter with history, with memory, with presence.

Protective gear is distributed. Suits, masks, visors, and layered gloves are provided. Tools are laid out on sanitized trays. A team of six is assigned to the first operation, three to dig, two to document, and one to oversee.

City officials from Sanitation and the Parks Department remain close, silently observant. They've signed off on every detail, but the emotional cost is not lost on them.

Andrew calls the team into a short circle. "We go slow. We honor sequence. No rush. No assumptions."

The group nods. Even Theo is uncharacteristically quiet.

Then, as the first layers of soil are carefully lifted from the trench's corner edge, the work resumes. It's deliberate, reverent, and irreversible. The Parks Department representative, a woman named Lila Torres, stands a few paces back, clipboard in hand. At first, she maintains professional detachment, eyes scanning the procedure, checking environmental compliance. However, as the remains of the first pine box become visible, its edges warped but intact, the outline is unmistakable. Her posture shifts.

Lila turns slightly, lowers her clipboard, and presses a hand over her mouth. For a moment, she tries to steady herself. But then her shoulders begin to shake. Tears stream down her cheeks before she has time to acknowledge them.

"I'm sorry," she murmurs, voice cracking. It's the kind of apology people make when tears come uninvited, when they feel the room noticing. "I wasn't ready for this."

No one responds with words. Meera steps beside her, a hand resting gently on her back. They stand there for a long breath, watching as the exposed edge of a forgotten life comes back into view.

The team proceeds with surgical care. The soil is removed centimeter by centimeter around the pine box, its structure compromised by age and moisture. As the lid collapses under its own weight, the interior is exposed. Cloth remnants, bone, and traces of leather shoes are revealed. Every artifact is documented, photographed, and then transferred into padded trays with gloved precision.

When the remains are lifted, it is done in silence. Each motion is coordinated. Gentle hands supporting the vertebrae, long bones, and the skull. What can be moved whole is moved whole. What cannot, is cupped gently, as though still living.

After each body is documented and its placement noted, it is returned to the same cavity from which it came. The team restores the pine fragments and brushes the surrounding earth back over with deliberate tenderness, careful to leave the site as undisturbed as possible.

Then, all fourteen coalition members, along with city officials and support staff, gather in a circle. No one speaks at first. Then Theo, holding a folded note, steps forward.

"This is continuity," he says softly. "We've asked questions of the dead. Today, they let us listen, and we're grateful."

The silence that follows is heavy and sacred. A moment held open.

Lila lowers her eyes, hands clasped. Meera places a single field marker at the site. Red flagged, labeled, and dated.

Only then do they step back.

Only then does the work continue.

Days pass. More remains are uncovered. Each one is documented, honored, and carefully returned to the ground. The process becomes a kind of dance. It moves through their arrival at the trench, quiet preparations, gentle footsteps around fragile outlines, and the soft murmur of notes recorded and verified.

Each team member knows their role, and the steps repeat with precision. There's a deep regard stitched into every motion. Metal trowels and soft brushes take the place of power tools; the hum of machinery has no place here. The brushing of soil from a fragment of cloth. The steadying of a collapsed ribcage. The pause before each final covering of soil and earth. Out of respect, they find themselves speaking less. The work is familiar, yes, but it never becomes commonplace. No one becomes numb.

Late on the sixth day, a new call rises from one of the central trenches. It's Julia.

"Stop," she says, her voice quiet and still firm. "This one's small."

Everyone freezes. Alain is the first to reach her side. The skeletal frame emerging from the soil is unmistakable. The delicate ribs, shorter limbs, and the arc of a developing skull. It's a child.

Silence ripples outward.

No one moves until Meera steps in, crouches, and nods once. Confirmation.

What follows transcends protocol. Science no longer drives them. This is more sacred. When the shroud is lifted, it's clear the body is that of a child. For a moment, no one moves. The procedures they've repeated all day fall away, replaced by something instinctive and collective. The team adjusts the schedule without a word, as though guided by something unspoken. One by one, each member of the team takes part. Whether it's lifting, supporting, or offering stillness, each movement is imbued with care. No one rushes. No one delegates. Each pair of hands holds the weight of a life cut short. Each gaze lingers just a little longer, acknowledging the absence and honoring it. In that moment, everyone becomes the pallbearer, and every gesture becomes a quiet vow. *You were here, and we see you now.*

The child's remains are returned to the earth with ceremony...and yet without spectacle. A circle forms again, this time unprompted. Hands are joined. Heads bow.

Theo, who usually speaks, says nothing. Even he knows the words would fall short.

Above them, gulls pass over in a quiet arc. The sun hangs low.

And beneath it all, the child rests. Seen, counted, and never again unknown.

By the close of the second week, the exhumation phase nears its end. The coalition has worked its way steadily through the decades, trench by trench, generation by generation. They began with the 1940s and concluded with those interred as recently as 2021, many from the pandemic years. With each excavation, the steps have grown more efficient, but never less reverent. The field logs are rich with layered data; the memory of each burial site preserved through presence.

Unexpectedly, the city observers who were initially positioned as monitors have joined the work in full. By the third day of exhumation, clipboards began to vanish, replaced with rubber gloves and face masks. One by one, representatives from Sanitation, Corrections, Public Health, and the Parks Department step into the field lines, shoulder to shoulder with the coalition team. There are no formal announcements. Just a quiet, evolving participation.

Lila Torres is among the first. Then comes Donovan from Sanitation, whose steady hands prove valuable when repositioning fragments. Marlene Chao, a nurse from Public Health, brings attention to detail when handling remains. Even Officer Luis Mercado, the correctional officer assigned to security, begins transporting sample kits to the mobile station without being asked.

By the final morning, every trench has known both scientist and steward. The lines have blurred between roles. Everyone here, by some quiet consensus, has become a caretaker.

Now the dead have presence. Once isolated by time and anonymity, they are counted by touch, by breath, and by name unknown.

That evening, back at the hotel, Meera, Andrew, and Theo gather in the quiet lounge area just off the lobby. The hum of the ice machine and the low clink of glassware at the far end of the bar are the only sounds heard as they drop into armchairs, weary and somehow still alert.

Theo stretches his legs and exhales. "Fourteen days on the island, and somehow it feels like both a month and a minute."

Andrew nods. "We haven't even started the data phase yet. What we collected and what we returned, it's going to take months to sequence, interpret, and publish."

Meera cradles her tea. "It's the 'return' part that stays with me tonight. The science matters, but the act of giving them back… That sticks with me."

Theo looks up. "You could feel it, couldn't you? Something happened after each reburial."

For a moment, they sit in silence.

"We will listen," Meera says at last. "As we always have. First to the soil. Then to the bones. And then to the model itself."

Theo raises his glass of Scotch. "To what answers come."

Andrew lifts his glass of ginger ale and vodka. "To the ones who waited to be found."

Meera lifts her chai cocktail, a smoky blend of bourbon, cardamom, and black tea, and joins them. "To whatever comes next."

They sit with their drinks for a while, the kind of silence that asks nothing and gives everything. The clink of ice. The muted hum of city life beyond the glass.

Then Meera shifts in her chair and glances toward Andrew. "What do you hear from Sonia and Junie?"

Andrew smiles, the kind of smile that softens everything else in his face. "Every day. Sonia's teaching schedule hasn't missed a beat. She's running her classes with that same blend of structure and soul. We talk each night after dinner, just to catch up. The other day, she told me her students were tracing family migration patterns across maps they drew themselves. She said it made them feel rooted, even if some of the routes were broken. She referred to it as 'roots grow in fractures.' That one stuck with me."

Theo whistles, impressed. "That's so her. Turning a hallway into philosophy."

"And Junie?" Meera asks.

Andrew's eyes light up. "She's taking more art classes. Said she wants to learn how to carve letters into stone. Last night she showed me a practice piece. She etched her own name into limestone. It was crooked, but proud. She asked if names still mattered if no one could pronounce them right."

Meera smiles. "What did you tell her?"

"That if names hold memory, then it doesn't matter who mispronounces it. Only who remembers it."

CHAPTER 20
TO SHIELD WHAT MATTERS

They return from Hart Island in quiet waves, dispersed across flights, trains, and slow ferry routes to their respective countries. No one speaks much during the travel. The weight of what they've seen and what they've done settles in different corners of their minds.

Andrew stares out the airplane window as the lights of Austin come into view below. He had taken the first flight out, even though it meant leaving Meera and Theo behind to catch the next one. They'd urged him to go. "Go home. Be with them," Meera had said, leaving no room for protest; but he hadn't argued. He took the earlier flight, realizing there was only room for one more. The gravity of Hart Island had settled deep, heavier than data or discovery, and the pull to see his family again outweighed everything else. Now, as the cabin dips into its final descent, he scrolls through photos of Junie on his phone and pauses on her latest drawing taped to their fridge. He knows Sonia will be awake when he gets home, lights low, waiting for him to walk through the door. The thought of home feels uncomplicated and welcoming.

Hours later, Meera's flight banks low over Austin as the sun sets, casting a gold wash across the Hill Country below. She closes the scientific journal in her lap. She hasn't turned a page in half an hour. Her mind keeps circling back to the moment the first body was returned to the earth. The hush, the ritual, the quiet shift in the air. This time, she's not passing through. She'll be based here for the foreseeable future, officially assigned to the U.S. research team as the work intensifies. She glances out the window, eyes tracing the unfamiliar skyline, wondering what Austin might teach her. The ground below is still foreign, but less so with each passing hour.

Theo sits beside Meera on the flight with a stack of loose papers balanced on his lap. They'd both agreed that Andrew should take the earliest flight home, but now, in the shared hush of the cabin, neither Meera nor Theo speaks much. Occasionally, Theo scribbles into the margin of his travel notebook, refining a soil lattice diagram that's been evolving in his head since the final sampling. He adds a note on residual mineral exchange and pauses, considering the implications. Meera glances over, recognizing the pattern of thought without needing to ask. She simply nods once, and they both return to their notes in silence.

On a separate flight heading east, Julia sits by the window, her forehead resting lightly against the cool plastic pane. Her thoughts moved past the protein markers and sequencing kits and focused on the dead. The man with the twisted wristwatch. The woman in the blue scarf who'd worn rosary beads in the grave. The child small, frail, and cradled in a rotting blanket as if still waiting for comfort. That one would not leave her. The child's empty ribs and soft jaw, barely formed, haunted the edges of her sleep each night on Hart Island. Julia clutches the edges of her scarf, eyes closed. The samples would tell their stories in time, she knows. Still, it's the memory of that child she carries home like a fingerprint pressed onto her chest unseen but never unfelt.

On a separate flight bound for Geneva, Alain sits quietly near the back of the cabin. His eyes drift over the cloud cover outside, but his thoughts remain grounded in the soil of Hart Island. He can still feel the heft of the shovel, the chill of the wind, the moment of silence that fell as the last of the bodies were lowered back into place. There is grief. Yet, underneath it, something else found a greater footing in his thoughts. Meaning. In all his years of environmental work, he has never felt this particular weight before. It's a combination of honor and responsibility. He touched history in the soil, in the fragile weight of the bones, and in the science itself.

Being there was more than theory and more than the writing on pages from a book. He exhales slowly, and for the first time in days, the corners of his mouth turn up in quiet resolve. Something good has taken place, and he has helped make it so.

Even as each team member carries the experience home in different ways, the work itself remains grounded. Steady and solemn. The samples are secure. Baseline data from undisturbed soil has been carefully sealed and logged. Days later, after reintroducing the bodies to the earth, they collect again, shovel by shovel, swab by swab, cataloging how the soil begins its transformation. Additional samples will be pulled in the months and years to come, forming a longitudinal record of what the earth chooses to remember, and what it lets go.

The process is methodical. However, this time, there are headlines. There are speeches. Andrew, Meera, and Theo step forward, reluctantly at first, to offer a record of what was accomplished on Hart Island and what is now being measured. They speak to global audiences, to scientific forums and press briefings, outlining how environmental composition and burial practices intersect in ways not previously quantified. Their words are careful, technical, and restrained. Designed to clarify, but nuance rarely survives translation. When Meera explains that "soil composition preserves biological signatures longer than expected," one outlet shortens it to "The soil remembers." Another headline calls it "The Language of the Earth." Soon, her phrasing circulates far beyond the data, reshaped by the world's appetite for meaning. Still, behind the microphones and away from the cameras, it is work that carries them forward.

Andrew finds himself standing at the edge of the temporary lab they've set up in the hospital's lower level, watching condensation form on the coolers that hold the Hart Island samples. He tracks each vial into the database, noting temperature, pH level, and trace organic shifts. There's a rhythm to it now. Data flows in columns. Observations stack like sediment.

Meera occupies a corner bench, cross-referencing spectral scans with soil chemistry records from earlier burial sites. Her chai sits forgotten and cold. The reintroduction of organic matter has already changed the soil's bacterial profile, and she's quietly noting every mutation, every early indicator of genome degradation or revival.

Theo, meanwhile, narrates his notes out loud to no one in particular, a stream of muttered thoughts as he syncs the new material with earlier samples pulled from the Netherlands. "Fungal bloom rising faster than expected... pH dipped but recovered... anaerobic threshold seems to align with..." He breaks off, tapping the edge of the desk, eyes narrowing. Then, abruptly, a tray clatters to the floor behind him. One of the sample carriers he had meant to re-rack, left slightly too close to the edge. Andrew and Meera look up in unison.

"It's fine," Theo mutters, already kneeling. None of the vials broke, but one is leaking condensation at an angle that draws his eye. "Actually, wait," he says. He lifts the tube and stares at it. "This wasn't supposed to show protein lift until day twenty."

Meera is at his side in seconds. She scans the chart on his tablet, then the tube. "It's accelerated. This one's ahead. Could be cross-contamination... or something else."

Theo exhales, equal parts frustration and awe. "Sometimes science just trips over itself and lands on something true."

None of them says it out loud, but each one knows this is the most delicate phase. It's no longer about finding data. It's about reading it properly.

The research room hums with subdued energy. Screens glow. Fridges open and close. Meera breaks the silence first by reaching over and placing one of her test trays next to Andrew's workstation. Their samples have begun to echo each other. Different sites. Same genetic drift.

No one is quite ready to name what they're seeing.

Elsewhere, New York is waking up to early summer. Sirens and birdsong intermingle. In here, they are deep in the aftermath, an aftermath filled with insight.

On the other side of the debate, the Shepherd's Stand Alliance remains vocal in its opposition. They call what happened in New York a desecration of hundreds of graves. In press releases and protest speeches, they question the coalition's ethics, warning that sacred boundaries have been crossed in the name of progress. At a vigil outside St. Mary's Cathedral, speakers hold placards marked with burial numbers and faded registry pages, reminders that anonymity does not erase dignity. Candles line the church steps as hymns rise through the crowd. In Albany, a state representative aligned with the Alliance introduces a motion to halt further testing on historical burial sites, citing cultural and spiritual violations.

A protest outside a downtown news station turns confrontational when demonstrators arrive in silence but escalate quickly as someone from the crowd demands an apology from Meera by name. Footage airs that evening of a woman being escorted away after trying to smear symbolic ashes across the station's glass doors.

Images from the protest, including banners, vigils, and quiet rows of lit candles, now occupy space in the public imagination. Slogans such as "The Dead Deserve Dignity" and "Science Must Respect the Sacred" appear on protest signs and hashtags spreading across social media. The noise continues with each news cycle, pressing the coalition into a defensive posture they had hoped to avoid.

In response, Sonia continues to serve as the coalition's public voice. With clarity and calm, she steps in to ask for patience and understanding, emphasizing that the Hart Island phase is only one part of a much broader inquiry. In a series of televised statements and published op-eds, she reminds the world that the goal is not disturbance but restoration, and that understanding how the balance between the living and the dead sustains the planet's biological health is essential. "Our work is about the continuity of life," she says at a Geneva press conference. "We study decomposition because it teaches us how ecosystems renew themselves. What we learn may one day help ensure healthier generations to come." Her message reframes the debate, giving the public a reason to listen. Headlines shift from outrage to cautious optimism. The world, stirred by fear and fascination, begins to soften its stance, turning bit by bit toward patience as it waits for answers.

That evening, at home in Austin, Sonia sets the table while Andrew plates up leftovers of chickpea stew and warm tortillas from HEB. Junie, now a little more attuned to the conversations around her, joins in with an ease that signals how much she's grown in the two years of the coalition research. She recites details from her day with curiosity and focus.

There's a new art project that explores storytelling through collage, a substitute math teacher who lets them play number trivia games, and a student council debate that stirred honest opinions in the classroom. She glances at Sonia between bites and says, "They talked about you at school today. Ms. Ramirez said you're helping the world remember things we forgot."

Sonia sets down the serving spoon and looks at Junie, her expression both proud and solemn. "That's kind of her to say. I hope that's what I'm doing. I also hope the world remembers what matters most, including kids like you having a normal day at school without cameras or microphones."

The rhythm of home returns, subtle and steady as the kitchen fills with the clatter of forks and the low hum of the Sonos speaker playing quietly from the windowsill. Beneath it all, Junie is listening, really listening, as her parents talk, her eyes flicking between them, absorbing more than she shares.

After Junie disappears down the hallway to prepare for bed, Sonia refocuses and exhales. "The principal pulled me aside today," she says. "They're nervous about the attention. A news van was parked outside this morning, and a few parents have started asking questions. Even just my name showing up on the broadcasts makes them uneasy. Angelina Eberly Elementary isn't used to that kind of visibility."

Andrew sets down his glass. "Are they asking you to step back?"

"Not yet," Sonia replies. "But you can feel it building. The district's trying to stay neutral, but the staff's uncomfortable."

Andrew runs a hand across his jaw, eyes drifting to the hallway. "Do you want to fight it? Or would it be a relief to let go of the spotlight for a bit?"

Sonia shakes her head slowly. "I don't know yet. I just know this isn't the kind of attention any of us asked for. Especially not Junie."

Sonia folds her napkin in her lap, then glances at Andrew. "I understand their point of view," she says. "I don't blame them for protecting their staff and students. But I also can't let the Alliance dictate the terms of this conversation. Not when we're this close to something real."

Andrew nods slowly. "You think the message is still getting through? With all the noise?"

"It has to," she says. "We're trying to help the world see what's really happening, how the same processes shaping the soil are shaping us. If the Alliance silences that, the outrage will become the story, and everything else—the science, the promise, the reason we began—will be lost."

Andrew reaches across the table and touches her hand. "Then we keep going. Carefully and visibly at the same time."

She squeezes his fingers, grateful.

They fall into silence again, listening to the water run in the bathroom sink and the soft creak of the floorboards as Junie moves around. Outside, the crickets chirp like nothing has changed at all.

The illusion of normalcy fades the next morning. As Sonia and Junie walk toward the school entrance, a pair of local reporters step out from the sidewalk, microphones lowered but cameras visible. One calls out politely, asking if Sonia can comment on the growing controversy. She keeps her gaze forward, tightening her grip on Junie's hand.

A staff member immediately approaches, ushering them through the doors. The district had promised to keep media off campus, but managing curiosity proves harder than expected.

Inside the hallway, Junie looks up at her mother. "Why were they filming us?"

"They're just doing their jobs," Sonia says, crouching to meet her eyes. "But it's not your job to talk to them. You just go be a kid, okay?"

Junie nods and hugs her tight before heading down the hall.

In her office, Sonia's hands are still trembling. She closes the door, lowers the blinds, and sinks into her chair. Outside, the muffled rhythm of morning announcements filters through the wall. She exhales slowly, knowing this won't be the last time their world brushes against the noise outside.

A few minutes later, Sonia opens a blank document and begins typing deliberately, carefully choosing each word. She drafts her resignation letter in quiet, steady strokes. She wants to shield the school from the noise that has begun to gather around her name. As she types, a memory drifts to the surface. It was her second year at the school when a quiet boy named Oscar refused to speak to anyone for weeks. Only after Sonia brought in a shoebox of rocks from her weekend hike, each one with a story attached, did Oscar reach out, pick up a smooth white stone, and whisper that it looked like the one from his grandmother's backyard. That was the day he began talking again. That was the day she understood that teaching meant helping others find their voice. And now, she realizes that calling has taken a different form.

She will not allow the circus outside to compromise the education, safety, and compassion within these walls. Angelina Eberly Elementary deserves room to breathe and teach without distraction. While she wholeheartedly believes in the coalition's mission, she refuses to be the wedge that divides a school from its community.

She prints the letter, signs it with a steady hand, and places it in an envelope.

By noon, it's on the principal's desk.

The following morning, the district releases a written statement on Sonia's behalf. It is brief and measured, but unmistakably hers.

"Today, I submitted my resignation to Angelina Eberly Elementary. This decision was my own. The school and its staff have been unwavering in their support, and I want to protect that. Classrooms should be places of discovery and belonging, not distraction or spectacle. I ask that all attention now turn away from this campus and its students.

I will continue my work with the coalition and the pursuit of scientific understanding, but I do so apart from the school community to shield what matters most."

By midday, the statement circulates across local news outlets. A few cameras linger at the school gate before moving on, and the story begins to lose momentum. Sonia spends the afternoon boxing up the contents of her classroom, her dignity intact, her purpose clearer than ever.

At Dell Children's, news of Sonia's resignation reaches the lab before the team quickly. Meera looks up from her tablet and sets it aside as Andrew walks in, shoulders tight, eyes distant.

"I read the statement," she says softly.

Theo swivels his stool toward them. "She handled it perfectly. Took control of the story before anyone else could."

Andrew nods but doesn't answer right away. He sets his coffee down, staring at the steam. "She shouldn't have had to," he finally says. "None of this should've touched her or the school."

Meera folds her arms on the table. "It was the only way to quiet it. The Alliance got their headlines, but they'll move on. They always do."

"Yeah," Theo says quietly. "They'll find something new to shout about next week."

Andrew exhales and looks out the lab window, the reflection of morning light dull in the glass. "She did the right thing," he says at last. "She pulled the noise off the kids and put it on herself. That takes more strength than most people ever see."

No one speaks after that. Typing on keyboards fills the silence as the team drifts back to their work. They continue processing, still moved, but resolved to keep going.

Later that afternoon, the three of them log onto a secure video call with coalition partners from across the globe. The screen fills with familiar faces, scientists from Tokyo, Amsterdam, São Paulo, and Nairobi. New delegates from Chile, South Korea, and Jordan have also joined. The coalition is growing. The questions are growing faster.

As greetings settle and screens stabilize, Meera shares her screen to reveal the latest sequencing results. "This is from the post-burial samples. Day seventeen," she says. "We're beginning to see expansions in complexity. Replication patterns that weren't there before."

Andrew adds, "Several of the protein markers we'd tagged in earlier controls have begun to display new bonding structures. Some of it resembles microbial behavior, but we're also seeing unexpected genomic bridges."

Theo chimes in from his corner. "It's not just recovery. It's convergence. These fragments are behaving more like networks that relics of the past."

The chat window on the call lights up with questions, observations, and excitement.

A researcher from Kenya asks, "Are you saying we're seeing cooperative activity across genetic remnants?"

"Yes," Meera confirms. "More than we anticipated. The New York soil is doing something remarkable. We don't know yet whether the process is stable or volatile, but the early signs suggest reactivation, metabolic patterns emerging in microbial communities we thought were dormant."

The screen goes quiet as the gravity of that statement settles in.

Then, a voice from Brazil announces, "We need to replicate this in our own conditions."

A new delegate from South Korea leans forward. "We may have access to archival soil near temple burial grounds. It could provide a clean comparison if local officials agree."

From Chile, a soft-spoken researcher adds, "We're working with communities near Atacama. Desert conditions give us a different lens. We'll need special protocols, but the isolation might reveal something even more fundamental."

A Jordanian microbiologist, joining the call for the first time, offers a nod. "We've begun early prep for controlled trials near ancient Nabatean sites. No disturbance yet. It's just observation."

"That's the right approach," Andrew says. "Let's map out a coordinated sequence schedule. We'll send out the primer kit revisions by the end of the week."

Around the world, the coalition nods in unison. The next phase is beginning.

CHAPTER 21
LEGACY MADE VISIBLE

The coalition gathers again virtually, their grid of faces spanning continents and time zones. It has been several months since the Normandy samples were collected and cataloged. Since then, French laboratories have been working steadily, their protocols meticulous, their analysis slow but revealing. The samples taken from the battlefields as well as those samples taken from the surrounding cliffs, fields, farmland, and urban settings within two kilometers of the original soil samples continue to yield traces of genetic material.

Camila opens the call with a recap, her tone both energized and reverent. As she speaks, a hush falls over the group from the quiet awe that has begun to accompany these discoveries. When she finishes, a pause lingers, until Dr. Nikhil Patel in Pune unmutes.

"I find myself thinking of our soil as a kind of manuscript," he says. "Each generation writes over the last, but the traces remain. What does it mean to live on land that carries those revisions beneath our feet?"

From Amsterdam, Dr. van Dalen adds, "There is something both humbling and unsettling about seeing molecular structures retain coherence beyond their expected timeline. It implies continuity, and perhaps, obligation."

Dr. Ishikawa from Tokyo nods solemnly. "In Shinto tradition, objects such as tools, places, and even land can hold spirit, or kami. This is not far from that. Perhaps the science is beginning to articulate what our ancestors sensed intuitively."

Camila folds her arms, thoughtful. "Maybe. But what we're measuring isn't spirit. It's transmission. Molecular residues that may influence early neurological formation. The language overlaps, but the mechanisms are what matter. If we can understand how ecological contact supports infant development, we can help prevent those deficits before they start."

Camila pauses for a moment and then continues, "That's what we're up against, isn't it? Explaining the data while also translating the quiet respect. What we're seeing is not just residual matter from the past. These aren't degraded strands or lifeless shadows of DNA. There's movement. There's repetition. Some of the sequences we detected in different plots are near-perfect echoes of each other, right down to the anomaly markers."

Theo nods, unmuting. "It's as if the soil itself is transmitting the material, or the patterns somehow. The patterns aren't just persistent, they seem to be propagating. Like drift, but with a level of fidelity that suggests something more deliberate, almost engineered."

A moment of silence follows. No one wants to be the first to make a claim too big to defend.

Andrew finally speaks. "Has there been any sign of degradation over time? Any tapering of signal strength in the older samples?"

"None," Camila says. "The earliest samples, even those exposed to weather and farming, still exhibit the same intensity. Even the newer samples appear consistent. We're not seeing a decay curve. If anything, it's a flat line."

"That's statistically unlikely," Meera says, leaning in. "Environmental noise alone should introduce some variability. But we're not seeing that. Which means either our testing methods are too narrow or the material is resisting entropy."

Theo attempts a smile. "Or the soil is magical. That's still on the table, right?"

Andrew lifts his glass in a mock toast. "Always."

They pause, sharing that rare camaraderie that only scientists at the edge of discovery understand. It's a mix of awe, disbelief, and the gnawing responsibility to be right.

Meera continues, "We have to consider that the material is either self-replicating, or it is being influenced by something in the environment we haven't identified yet. Maybe fungal networks, maybe microbial symbionts. But something is maintaining or reproducing these sequences."

"They're clustered," Camila adds. "They're not evenly distributed, which suggests a vector."

Peter chimes in for the first time. "Could it be the burial customs themselves? Across cultures, mourners often added traces of their own bodies—hair, nails, blood, even ash—to the graves of relatives. Over centuries, those cumulative offerings might have altered the surrounding biology, embedding a record of both the dead and the living."

Theo smiles. "So, what you're saying is the soil has culture."

There's a pause.

Then Meera breaks into laughter. "Put that on a coffee mug."

Camila grins. "Or a grant proposal."

Andrew is quiet for a moment, then asks, "What are our next steps? We can't explain this yet, but we also can't ignore it."

Theo replies, "We dig. Literally. Expand the study sites in new directions. We already have inquiries pending for the Ainu burial forest in northern Hokkaido, the salt-preserved catacombs in southern Italy, and a series of rural hamlets in western Ghana where oral histories point to centuries of intact burial rituals.

We need environmental contrast too. We should compare arid zones, alpine, and floodplains. I've asked for access to a glacier-adjacent graveyard in Yukon, and Meera mentioned a terraced site in Himachal Pradesh known for seasonal washout but deep cultural continuity. The idea is to broaden our sample environments beyond Western contexts and see whether the same genomic signatures are appearing under dramatically different ecological and anthropological conditions. Expand the study sites. Compare soil samples from known sterile environments such as industrial parks, parking lots, and recently deforested zones. See if the signal holds up outside ritual or inhabited areas."

"We revisit the burial records," Meera adds. "Cultural overlays, recurring rituals, even oral histories. If the soil is holding onto something, we need to understand what was put there in the first place."

Andrew nods. "Alright. Let's formalize the next phase. We re-test Normandy and add at least four more locations. We'll include control sites that should, by all accounts, show nothing."

Peter volunteers, "I can get clearance for some sites in rural Sweden. Very little agricultural interference and minimal burial rituals for centuries. If we find anything there, it's systemic and not just drift."

Camila agrees to liaise with the French labs for expedited sequencing. Meera starts drafting the metadata schema for cultural indexing. Theo updates the shared database to accommodate multiple comparative layers.

Andrew glances at the clock in the corner of the screen, then clears his throat. "Before we break, I want to raise something else. Theo, you mentioned pressure-testing the model. How far have we taken that?"

Theo nods, already pulling up a tab. "We've been collecting external validations since late last quarter. The labs Meera contacted in India, both in Hyderabad and Kerala, ran full-cycle replicative testing. Then the Soil Research Consortium in Pune agreed to model layering with cultural overlays. Their datasets tracked within our predictive margin."

Meera jumps in, eyes bright. "More importantly, they used independent sequencing protocols, different reagents, and different soil filters. The replication rate remained above ninety-two percent. That's well within our tolerance band."

Andrew raises an eyebrow. "So, no wild deviations?"

"None that break the model," she replies. "They each showed a slight delay in signal emergence. It's probably due to soil pH and particulate density, but the patterns aligned."

Theo adds, "Dr. van Dalen came through as well. His colleagues at Wageningen ran side-by-sides with data from Oslo, and both sites confirmed lateral drift with anomalous repetition markers. Same clustering. Same structural encoding."

Camila exhales softly. "So, the model's holding. Not just theoretically. Empirically."

"Exactly," Theo says. "Pressure testing validated the framework, reinforcing that what we see isn't an anomaly. It's a pattern, and it's stable."

Andrew leans back, letting that settle. "Then it's time we start saying that out loud, outside of our peer calls. We need to publish it."

Meera nods. "I'll finalize the cross-lab summary. We'll lead with the Indian and Dutch validations. The French data will still serve as the narrative base."

Theo's voice is quietly confident. "The world's going to have questions. We need to be ready with answers."

Andrew nods. "We will be."

That evening, Meera and Theo arrive at Andrew and Sonia's house just after dusk, arms full of takeout and annotated notebooks. The kitchen is warm and smells faintly of roasted garlic and cumin from an earlier prep that Sonia decided not to serve but let perfume the house anyway. The table is already cleared except for a single candle and Sonia's laptop, its screen glowing faintly with draft language for the coalition's first formal public statement.

Junie pads into the kitchen in fuzzy socks, her eyes lighting up when she sees Meera. Without hesitation, she wraps her arms around Meera's waist in a sleepy hug. "You're here more now," she murmurs. Meera smiles and kisses the top of her head. "I like being here."

Junie then grins at Theo, who wiggles his eyebrows and pulls a wrapped fortune cookie from his pocket like it's treasure. "For my favorite nighttime ninja," he whispers. She giggles and pockets it, then offers a sleepy wave to Sonia and Andrew before disappearing down the hallway, still smiling.

"Was that your last cookie?" Sonia asks Theo, raising an eyebrow.

"I may have a backup stash," he grins. "Junie's been training me in the art of covert snack diplomacy."

They all laugh, grateful for the levity.

Andrew pours glasses of wine while Sonia plates up small bowls of mango salad and sticky rice, a nod to comfort more than cuisine. They eat casually; papers pushed aside for the moment.

"Can we just admit that we've all been dreaming about soil?" Theo says as he chews. "I caught myself narrating sample comparisons in my sleep."

"I woke up quoting pH charts," Meera admits.

Sonia chuckles. "I think I heard Andrew mumbling 'genomic harmonics' at two a.m."

"Not possible," Andrew replies with mock indignation. "I'm strictly a nighttime entropy philosopher."

They linger over their plates a few minutes longer before the conversation shifts toward the work.

Sonia clears a space on the table and opens the laptop wider. "Alright. Let's get serious."

Andrew lays out hard copies of the modeling forecast. "We're going to have to be careful here," he says. "We can't overwhelm people with data, but we can't shy away from what the scenarios predict either."

Theo flips to the section marked SCENARIO THREE and taps the margin. "This is the one they'll fixate on. Rewilding protocols and biome reactivation. It's going to sound radical."

"Because it is," Sonia says. "But it's also testable, and we've already started. Hart Island gave us the pilot. We just haven't called it that yet."

Meera nods. "The predictive model held in all three scenarios, but scenario three showed the highest long-term rebalancing. Lower genomic dropout, stronger microbial integrity, and fewer anomalies in secondary decay layers."

Andrew flips a page. "Scenario one was the baseline. Do nothing and maintain modern entombment. It continues the decline."

"Scenario two," Theo adds, "is a return to traditional decomposition. Some gain, but not consistent across regions. Cultural resistance and regulatory hurdles."

Sonia speaks firmly and with inquiry. "Scenario three, the controlled reintegration model. That's the one the projections show as most promising, right? If those outcomes hold, it could finally give the public something hopeful to grasp."

They fall into a thoughtful silence, eyes resting on the same document.

"It's not just about decay rates," Meera says finally. "It's about the earth

contributing to the repair. All of us deciding whether we want to participate in that memory or isolate ourselves from it."

Theo lifts his glass. "Then let's make that the heart of the statement.
Not just science. Responsibility."

Andrew nods. "We frame it carefully. We say what we know. We say
what we don't. And we offer a path."

Sonia opens a new document. "Then let's write it."

Her fingers hover over the keyboard before she begins to type. The
silence in the room shifts away from the anticipation and toward the
gravity of circumstance. Sonia's mind flits briefly to her students, to
Junie's quiet resilience, and to the mothers she's spoken with at community centers who don't have the language to describe what they sense is
wrong in the environment around them. She feels the weight of this
moment more as a mother trying to thread caution through hope.

She wants the message to land softly without losing its urgency. To
avoid blame but not dodge accountability. Most of all, she wants it to do
what science often struggles to do in public. Make people feel invited and
not dismissed. She breathes in slowly and asks Andrew to join her so they
can write this together.

She types as Andrew voices the science, translating it into something
the public can digest. The rhythm of keys is a soft undertone to their
gathered focus. When they finish the first section, she reads it aloud.

"Around the world, doctors and pediatric researchers have observed a
concerning rise in birth defects and developmental anomalies. Many of
them appear during the formative years of childhood. While the causes
are still being studied, a growing body of evidence suggests environmental factors may contribute. Something in the soil and earth around us
has changed.

"For the past year, an international coalition of scientists has been
studying soil samples from around the world, testing for signs of genetic
memory, decay, and drift. We've found both unexpected and promising
results. Some soil systems, particularly those associated with historical
burial and cultural sites, continue to exhibit active genomic patterns. By
'genomic patterns,' we mean identifiable sequences of genetic material,
fragments of DNA or RNA, that remain stable in the soil. They often

mirror each other across locations. These patterns do not degrade with time; in some cases, they appear to replicate.

"This is not a declaration of danger. It is a call to attention.

"The earth appears to be retaining more biological memory than previously understood. Our models have shown stable persistence and potential propagation of genetic fragments within soil ecosystems through controlled studies in France, the Netherlands, India, and the United States.

"Our data supports three future pathways. One continues the current burial practices unchanged. One returns to natural decomposition. The third, now under active testing, involves reintegrating entombed remains into living soil through biome restoration and rewilding protocols. This third path shows the greatest promise for restoring genomic stability in affected regions.

"We are not asking the world to choose today. We are asking the world to look."

After hearing Sonia voice the joint message, Meera pauses, processing the cadence of the statement. "It's good," she says. "Strong. Grounded. Still, I think we should also explain *why* this association between earth and body matters. We're asking people to care about something invisible. So, we need to give them a way in."

She pulls her notebook closer. "Think about how genetically identical plants can grow differently depending on the microbes in the soil or the trace minerals in the water. The same seed, different outcome, because the environment rewrites the expression."

Theo nods slowly. "The same principle applies to people."

"Exactly," Meera says. "Environmental factors can upregulate or silence genes, especially in developing embryos. Recall the example we discussed a few months ago. A mother's nutrition or stress during pregnancy can affect the child's long-term health by altering gene expression. This is similar to that."

Sonia begins typing again, murmuring as she goes: "The land isn't passive. It interacts with us quietly, chemically, and generationally. If it retains molecular traces of what came before, then those traces influence what follows. We live within that continuum."

The following day, the full coalition reconvenes.

Each member logs into the secured video platform with a digital copy of Sonia's memorandum already in hand. In the hours leading up to the call, inboxes across five continents lit up with final review notes. Camila stayed late in São Paulo to review the translated version with a team of legal scholars and civil planners. In Pune, Dr. Patel conferred with two colleagues on how to frame the findings in a culturally sensitive way for a press inquiry he knew would come. In Amsterdam, van Dalen had reviewed soil drift overlays until midnight, triple-checking every margin of error.

Even Ishikawa in Tokyo, normally reserved, circulated a brief reflection to the group hours earlier. A single paragraph bridging traditional belief with empirical science, quietly urging courage.

They arrived at the call informed and invested. Each participant lived through the weight of the findings in their own soil, their own language. They share more than the science. They share the proper narrative.

There's a solemn energy in their virtual room, anticipatory and grounded. This is a turning point.

Andrew opens the meeting. "You've all had time to read the draft. We're not here to workshop language. We're here to weigh its release."

Camila nods. "The tone is careful. Thoughtful. It presents the science clearly without dramatizing the risk."

"I agree," says Peter. "It doesn't overreach, and it avoids panic. It's very effective at inviting observation."

From the Tokyo node, Dr. Ishikawa speaks. "The data may be complex, but the message is human. People can follow this. They need to."

Meera glances around the screen. "This is what we've built toward. Clear datasets which invite a shift in understanding. The statement frames it well. It also frames our responsibility."

Theo adds, "If we wait for perfect consensus, we'll be explaining ourselves too late. We have replication. We have confirmation. And we now have language that brings others in. It's time."

A brief silence falls again, followed by small nods from every corner of the digital room.

Andrew lifts his gaze. "Then we have consensus?"

One by one, voices confirm.

"Yes."

"Approved."

"I support it."

"Release it."

Andrew exhales. "Then we move forward. Today."

Before the call ends, Camila taps her microphone to recenter everyone's attention. "We're ready in São Paulo. Three pilot sites. Former burial grounds that are now redesigned as living gardens. Each integrates ecological thresholds, cultural access, and community oversight. We've cleared the final regulatory barriers. What was theory is now policy."

Meera sits forward. "Will the release of the statement jeopardize local support?"

Camila shakes her head. "Quite the opposite. It's been quiet because there was nothing public to react to. Once this goes live, the media attention will force the next conversation. The benefit is that now we're ready for it."

Theo nods thoughtfully. "You're saying it's no longer a hypothetical. Legacy gardens are real enough to protect." He pauses, then adds, "Just last week, a woman wrote that her grandfather's grave will become part of the garden. She called it a kind of reconciliation. That word stayed with me."

"Exactly," Camila says. "And once the public hears the science, I believe we'll find more cities ready to listen."

Let's make it official," Andrew says.

Camila smiles. "It already is."

The screens blink dark one by one, leaving the reflection of the last image. Green plots on the São Paulo map are mirrored in the glass. Outside Andrew's window, sunlight shines through. What was once a theory now waits in the soil.

CHAPTER 22
LET GO OF THE STONE

The statement is released at eight GMT on Tuesday. Translated and posted selectively by coalition partners and research institutions, it appears first in targeted regions. Within an hour, it begins trending across those networks, carrying a single question that headline writers lift from it.

"Does the Earth remember us?"

That line becomes the anchor.

Among the initial release regions, reactions are swift and polarized. In the United States, major networks split along predictable lines. Public health officials express cautious interest, while pundits argue over whether this is science or spiritualism dressed in lab coats.

In Canada, the conversation is gentler, more academic. University panels convene within days. CBC runs a town hall with Indigenous leaders and soil scientists discussing the resonance between traditional knowledge and emerging research. National response is characterized by a quiet openness, a wait-and-see posture that leans toward engagement.

In France, where the soil studies originated, the national response is subdued and thoughtful. Le Monde publishes a special feature titled *La Mémoire des Sols*, "The Memory of Soil," and profiles Camila's work in São Paulo alongside Meera's findings in Kerala. Television coverage is minimal, maintaining a respectful tone. Interviews with French ecologists and philosophers highlight how the concept of genetic memory in soil resonates with longstanding continental ideas about land, death, and continuity. While the French Ministry of Research stops short of endorsement, it announces funding for a formal inquiry into the coalition's claims.

In Asia, early attention centers on India, with echoes in neighboring cultural and academic circles. In India, Meera is invited to speak on *Doordarshan* in both Hindi and English. Viewership spikes as her appearance is shared across platforms, interspersed with clips of local farmers and Ayurvedic practitioners echoing her observations about the soil. Buddhist scholars in South Korea and Japan weigh in, drawing connections between ancestral dignity and the coalition's findings, especially the idea that the land holds karmic imprint and legacy. In Kyoto, a Zen monastery hosts a discussion series titled *The Living Earth*, blending modern soil science with sutras on impermanence and rebirth.

Across much of Africa, where burial practices already reflect a living relationship with soil, the reaction carries a reserved respect. In Ghana, researchers begin a study on the ancestral groves near Kumasi, where elders have long spoken of land that "remembers blessings and betrayals." Kenya's National Museums Service collaborates with local communities in Kisumu to document traditional burial wisdom alongside sample collection. In both countries, emphasis is placed on community consultation and the spiritual dimensions of land care.

As the first week unfolds, interest spreads southward. South Africa's Environmental Affairs Ministry formally asks to join the coalition as an observer and begins reviewing possibilities for a legacy garden pilot within the Eastern Cape, where Xhosa burial rites already emphasize biological reintegration. The South African Broadcasting Corporation (SABC) runs a series titled *The Soil Beneath*, spotlighting rural communities whose relationship to the land blurs the lines between biology, culture, and inheritance. The response is cautious, deeply rooted in cultural alignment.

South America, Brazil in particular, embraces the announcement more fully. The framework Camila helped establish in São Paulo becomes a reference point, especially as it weaves modern scientific methodology with long-standing Afro-Brazilian spiritual traditions tied to land and ancestral veneration. In Salvador and Recife, community leaders note that the idea of the soil holding memory aligns with the Candomblé belief that spirits return to the earth as a form of continuity and care.

By week's end, the coalition is fielding dozens of inquiries from universities, NGOs, and cultural ministries seeking guidance or collaboration.

For the first time, the conversation feels shared. From villages and temples to laboratories and government halls, the message has sparked something rare: a quiet convergence of curiosity and care. Though ideologies differ and skepticism remains, the world is listening—wondering whether the earth holds more than we thought.

The following Tuesday, the coalition regroups on a secure video call. The mood is electric and charged with a quiet intensity.

Andrew opens. "We've never seen engagement like this. Not for something this… nuanced."

Meera nods. "The scientists aren't alone in their curiosity and interest. It's farmers, teachers, spiritual leaders. People are trying to make sense of this with the frameworks they already have. And for once, those frameworks are compatible."

Theo looks directly into his camera. "I got three interview requests in twenty-four hours. Two from soil science journals. One from *Vogue*, if you can believe that. They're running a feature on sustainability and burial reform."

A few smiles ripple across the screen, and there's a shared recognition among them. The story is spreading beyond academia, crossing into culture. Their work has slipped into the public conversation, and that changes the tone of everything that follows.

Camila adds, "São Paulo city council wants to fast-track the legacy garden permits. I thought I'd be fighting for two years. Now they're asking how quickly we can begin public education programs."

Dr. Ishikawa, serene as ever, smiles faintly. "I was asked to speak at a Shinto university in Kyoto. They said the science reminds them of the oldest prayers, that memory is always with us and not behind us."

Peter joins from Amsterdam. "Several municipalities and cemetery boards are reaching out. They're asking what a transition to 'semi-active soil spaces' would even require. Permits, oversight, community input—the whole thing. That phrase didn't exist two months ago."

Sonia listens quietly, then speaks. "We need to stay grounded. This is spreading fast. That's a gift, but also a risk. We need consistency. Clarity."

Andrew agrees. "We set the tone early. If the science gets twisted into mysticism, we lose credibility. However, if we ignore the emotional resonance, we lose people."

Meera nods slowly. "So, we walk the line. Invite them in while staying anchored."

Andrew shifts slightly in his chair, then gestures toward his screen. "Now that we're all excited, I want to circle back to the Normandy data. The samples we reviewed two meetings ago."

Meera straightens. "Yes, I've been thinking about it constantly. The sequences we pulled from the post-burial plots... they're still expressing."

Camila tilts her head. "You mean persisting," she says in a statement of correction.

"No," Meera says. "I mean replicating. Either the material is self-replicating, or it's being influenced by something in the environment. Possibly microbial symbionts. Something is maintaining these sequences."

"And they're clustered," Camila reminds the group. "They're not evenly distributed, which suggests a vector. Some mechanism of transfer or amplification. The control soil doesn't show the same pattern. Yet, the soil where reintroduction occurred is patterned. Spatially organized, like a slow-moving bloom."

Theo murmurs, "So it's not just memory. It's activity."

Meera nods. "Exactly. Something is happening. The soil isn't static. It's communicating, maybe even adapting. We need to explore whether these clusters correspond to microbial colonies or environmental gradients."

Dr. Ishikawa jots notes. "Could this be biotically mediated transmission? Fungal threads? Root systems?"

"Or weather systems," Theo adds. "Or insects. If there's a biological courier, we need to know."

Sonia says sharply, "Then Normandy is no longer a pilot, it's our live field lab. Let's treat it that way. We should monitor Hart Island for the same."

Theo picks up on Sonia's point. "Hart Island is different, though. It's not just a soil reintroduction site. It's a layered record of marginalized death. If the patterns start showing up there too, especially in the newer strata, that could mean this process isn't ancient. It's current."

Meera pauses, then adds quietly, "And if it's current, it's transferable. We may be looking at a feedback loop between the living and the buried. A cycle that never fully broke."

Andrew looks toward his camera. "Which means whatever's happening underground isn't just residue. It's inheritance. If the soil is still participating in biological exchange, then what future generations draw from it — food, water, microbiome — could carry echoes of what came before."

Camila exhales slowly. "So, the question isn't just whether the Earth remembers us," she says. "It's how that memory continues."

Andrew nods slowly. "The post-burial samples from Hart haven't been fully sequenced yet. We prioritized Normandy because of the cleaner environmental controls. We can shift resources if it's necessary."

"I'll coordinate with the New York team," Julia offers. "We'll run comparative sequencing on the reintroduced plots and the untouched control lots. If replication is happening in both locations under different climates and burial histories, that's a data point the world can't ignore."

Camila glances at her notes. "Let's add São Paulo to that. I can push the local council to allow a pre-study phase in one of the undeveloped zones. Early soil pulls only. No public notice yet."

Dr. Ishikawa folds his hands. "We'll do the same in Kyoto. Quiet sampling. Temple grounds only. We'll frame it as a cultural biodiversity survey if we need to buy time."

Meera's voice is resolute. "We don't just need replication. We need triangulation. If we can show this isn't environmental noise or cultural artifact, and these clusters emerge in different geographies with different microbial lineages, then we prove something more than persistence. We prove pattern. Direction."

Andrew looks around at the screen full of thoughtful, blinking eyes.

"Alright. Normandy, Hart Island, São Paulo, Kyoto. That's our priority set. Four continents. One hypothesis."

Theo smiles faintly. "Let's see if the Earth says the same thing in four languages."

Just then, Meera's phone chimes.

Everyone pauses. Theo and Andrew, seated across from her at the lab's central worktable, both turn instinctively to look at Meera in real time, no screen needed. The others on the call shift their gaze to her thumbnail.

She lifts the phone and stares at the screen. Her expression doesn't change immediately. Just a small, drawn-in breath that catches Theo's and Andrew's attention across the lab table. She blinks once, then again, as if trying to reprocess what she's just read.

Theo leans forward. "Meera?"

The screen is silent. The remote participants watch in muted suspense.

She slowly sets the phone down on the table. "It's the cross-lab results," she says, voice tight. "Pune, Wageningen, and Oslo all just submitted."

A brief silence.

"Independent verification of the predictive model..."

Another pause, long enough for Sonia to sit up straighter. Her hand instinctively moves to her notepad.

"Confirmed."

A pause of silence.

Andrew's voice calls out a little louder than expected. "Confirmed?"

Meera nods. "All three labs replicated the key markers across different soil compositions and climate profiles. The algorithm holds. The decay curves match. And within the replication window we proposed, they saw the same bloom rate within our acceptable margin."

"So, the model is no longer a theory," Sonia states almost as a question.

"It's a framework," Meera says. "One the global scientific community just accepted."

Theo whispers, almost reverently, "We have proof."

Andrew looks at him. "Proof of persistence, yes. But not yet proof of influence."

Meera nods slowly. "Exactly. We've shown that genetic fragments re-enter the biome and remain active. What we don't yet know is whether that activity reaches forward into the food chain, the microbial exchange, or the people who live on that land."

Camila's voice comes through the speaker. "Then that's the next step. The bridge between the dead and the living isn't symbolic anymore. It's measurable."

For a moment, no one speaks.

Andrew stretches back slightly in his chair and lets out a long breath. This is the start of something heavier. "I wasn't sure we'd ever get here," he says with a quiet voice. "I believed in it, sure. But having the data… It's like watching a theory grow lungs and start to breathe."

Meera gives a small nod without breaking her gaze from the table. "I used to tell myself it was enough just to ask the right questions. Now, though, we're answering them, and the answers are demanding things from us. Big things."

Theo, still blinking at the screen, lets out a soft laugh. "I thought I'd be thrilled. I guess I am, but I also feel like we just unlocked something that can't be put away again. No red button. No off switch."

Camila, speaking from São Paulo, steps in. "When I walked into that city council meeting last month, I expected resistance. Years of it. But they didn't argue. They welcomed it. They're calling it *restorative public ecology*. While that's amazing, it's also terrifying. We're not just theorizing. We're influencing public infrastructure."

Meera folds her arms, her voice steady and slow. "This means we're no longer scientists standing behind glass. We're part of the ecosystem now. The public has handed us trust and some fear, too. We owe them clarity." Shae pauses for a moment before continuing. "We owe them space to feel this."

Dr. Ishikawa's voice comes through the speaker with assurance. "I lit incense this morning for the responsibility. The more we know, the more sacred this becomes."

Theo looks over at Meera and Andrew in the lab. "Do you think we're ready for what comes next?"

Andrew doesn't answer right away. He looks at the papers scattered across the desk. The simulation charts are now obsolete in the face of real data.

"I think," he finally says, "we'll have to become the kind of people who are."

Theo snaps to attention. "We need to update the public statement. This changes everything."

Sonia nods. "We need to move quickly. The original statement was cautious by necessity. It was rooted in observation, but now we have replication. We have validation."

Camila adds, "It gives us the credibility to project forward and show that the forecast scenarios aren't speculative."

Meera opens her laptop. "I'll revise the language on the model's status. We'll add a preamble noting cross-lab verification and clarify that Scenario Three is now in early-stage confirmation."

Dr. Ishikawa looks into his camera. "We should include the margins of error and lab affiliations. Transparency will protect us from early mischaracterization."

Sonia agrees. "We lead with humility and avoid downplaying the weight of this. The world's listening now; so, we tell them what we know and what comes next."

It doesn't take long for Scenario Three to become the lightning rod.

In the United States and Canada, media coverage quickly polarizes. Talk radio hosts and digital influencers reduce the science to its most inflammatory premise: "They want us to dig up Grandma and toss her back into the dirt."

In contrast, the response across Europe and Asia, especially in countries with longstanding traditions of earth-based burial and ecological integration, is far more reverent. In Japan, Shinto priests and soil microbiologists appear side-by-side on national panels, interpreting Scenario Three as a rebalancing of human presence and planetary care. In India, editorialists draw parallels to Prithvi, the earth goddess, and call the findings "a scientific invitation to rejoin a sacred cycle."

Even in Germany and France, where public discussion remains cautious, religious and academic institutions are starting serious debates about changing cemetery practices to consider soil biology.

In a hillside monastery in South Korea, a Buddhist nun named Haejin kneels in the morning mist. Around her, monks, microbiologists, and grieving families gather in a circle, hands resting on the soil. Incense drifts above it, thin and deliberate. The prayers alternate between Korean and Sanskrit, with the language of science threaded quietly among them, phrases such as persistence, decay curve, and microbial bloom. Haejin calls it a prayer for balance. The ceremony airs live on Korean public television.

In Alberta, Canada, an Indigenous elder named Evelyn convenes a talking circle beneath a grove of whispering aspens. She passes a small pouch of tobacco to each participant, encouraging them to speak their truth to the land. Her voice is steady as she speaks of kitaskînaw, the living earth, and the stories that sleep beneath it. Young people nod quietly while older voices tremble, recalling family burial plots threatened by erosion and forgotten by bureaucracy. The moment is both cathartic and visionary. When someone asks what they should do next, Evelyn replies, "We start by caring for the ground that's already ours. Then we teach others to do the same."

On the outskirts of Kisumu, Kenya, a botanist named Dr. Wekesa introduces a new unit to his high school science class: Soil, Culture, and Continuity. Students sit under acacia trees and read oral histories of burial practices beside lab sheets showing genetic material extracted from soil samples. Wekesa invites elders from the Luo community to explain how burial mounds are layered with ecological knowledge. The students are mesmerized. Later, a girl named Atieno asks whether her grandmother's land might hold more than crops. Wekesa smiles. "It holds the instructions for life."

A global dialogue begins to unfold, but it is no longer just about what's possible.

It's about what people are willing to believe, and what they're willing to let go.

Elsewhere in the quiet hours following the coalition's major announcement, a private conversation opens between two of its members.

Alain reaches out to Meera personally, his message uncharacteristically hesitant but heartfelt. The coalition video calls were public, performative in a way. This is not. When they finally connect, his voice carries more weight than usual.

"I keep thinking about my father," he says. "My grandparents too. They're all buried in a cemetery just outside Marseille. I've visited them for decades. I planted lavender on the graves. It was always... memory. Stillness."

Meera listens with respect.

"And now," Alain continues, "I find myself wondering what it would mean to return them to the earth in a truer sense. Not sealed beneath stone but rejoined with the land. Intellectually, I understand the model. I believe the science. But emotionally?" He pauses. "It's grief all over again. Combined with something else. Maybe it's restoration."

Meera listens closely, then asks gently, "What do you think your father would say, if you told him what we've learned?"

Alain is silent for a moment, the question catching him off guard. "He was a scientist too, before he retired. Curious. Skeptical, always. More than that, he believed in renewal. He taught me to compost before I could ride a bike."

He gives a soft laugh. "He might call this poetic logic, but he'd listen. If he saw what I see, he'd want to be part of it. Even if it meant letting go of the stone above him."

Meera is quiet for a long moment, letting Alain's words settle. "In Kerala," she finally says, "my grandmother was buried behind the house. No casket. Just a woven mat and the mango tree above. Every time I walk that path, I wonder if the soil remembers her differently than we do."

She looks out the window of her office. "My family used to joke that the roots of that tree made the mangoes sweeter. Well, maybe it wasn't a joke."

Alain doesn't speak, and he doesn't need to.

"It's strange," Meera continues. "We've studied the science, written the algorithms, calibrated the decay curves, yet here I am, still imagining her in the soil, not gone, just... changed."

She hesitates, then adds, "Even now, when I look at the models, I can't help thinking of her. Those microbial exchange rates, the mineral uptake

—it's all data, yes, but it's also a story. Every data point traces a life returning to balance. That's what we've measured, and what we're still learning to feel."

She turns back to the screen. "This isn't just a shift in how we bury. It's a shift in how we remember. And maybe, how we belong."

Alain nods slowly. "The beauty is that the numbers agree. The carbon cycling and the biodiversity indices each echo what the old traditions always knew. When we open the ground to renewal, everything improves. The science proves it; faith affirms it."

CHAPTER 23
THE LIVING SYSTEM

The coalition call begins with the quiet symphony of people logging in from around the world. Chimes, notifications, and flickers of light and video feeds stabilize. Meera sits in the lab in Austin, flanked by Theo, Sonia, and Andrew, each positioned with a tablet or laptop. Behind them, the soft whir of lab equipment continues its ceaseless rhythm. Sonia, freshly untethered from her school commitments, now holds a more central role. Dell Children's media team has brought her on as a contract employee to ensure the hospital retains a hand in shaping the public narrative while also preventing any of her contributions from rendering future findings non-tangible for the institution. The hospital has a financial stake in what is learned from these experiments, especially if discoveries made through enriched soil yield new diagnostic tools or therapies. Sonia has leaned into the project with characteristic focus, reviewing data, designing new learning modules, and liaising with educators who are desperate for accurate, age-appropriate materials.

One by one, coalition members check in.

Dr. Kamara appears first, her feed showing a packed lecture hall in Sierra Leone. "We've had nonstop press interest since the burial soil results were published. The university is organizing a public symposium next week. I'll be speaking alongside a local imam and a traditional healer to address growing fears and encourage transparency."

From Kyoto, Dr. Shun Hamada logs in next. He's seated on a cushion in what looks like his home office, sunlight filtering through paper-paneled doors. "NHK ran a feature last night. It's prompted calls from Shinto scholars. Some were worried while others were merely curious. We've invited a group of them to tour our soil labs. There's cautious optimism."

Dr. Camila Velasquez joins from São Paulo, her background alive with activity. "The city council approved our proposal for extended soil sampling at burial sites, urban green spaces, and even playgrounds. We're drafting new consent forms for families, trying to balance respect with urgency. The press has been aggressive, but there's strong public interest."

A few moments later, Dr. Yusuf Farah in Nairobi offers a brisk nod. "We've had two national news segments in the last week. I joined a panel discussion with religious leaders and geneticists. Lots of tension, but also curiosity. We're initiating soil comparisons across schoolyards and unmarked graves."

As the meeting proceeds, each update weaves another thread into the tapestry of global reaction. It's a mixture of concern, resistance, hope, and cooperation.

Back in Austin, Meera facilitates the discussion. "Thank you all. Before we move into today's agenda, I want to acknowledge the pace and scale of this moment. We started as a quiet hypothesis in a single lab. Now, we're steering an international dialogue grounded in science while touching belief, history, and grief."

"Which makes our next decisions even more critical," Andrew says. "The next stage moves past the data. It's about trust."

Sonia nods and adds, "And learning. People are hungry for under-standing, but they're knowingly scared. We need to help teachers, doctors, and community leaders translate what we're finding. Otherwise, it'll be the loudest voices, often the least accurate, that shape the narrative."

Andrew taps a few keys to bring up a shared presentation. "Let's start with the updated soil degradation models, as well as the solid transmission data. We've received continuing updates from the New York labs regarding Hart Island. The legacy signal appears to be rebounding quite measurably. Signal strength, once thought to be dissipating beyond recovery, is now registering at levels six to eight percent above baseline from six weeks ago. It's far too early for meaningful conclusions, but the consistency across multiple quadrants is worth noting."

Meera continues the discussion by offering, "More intriguing, early botanical assays show that surrounding plant roots already exhibit altered gene expression patterns, particularly in stress response and cell wall biosynthesis pathways. These changes align with previously observed reactions in Normandy, where genetically stable plants still showed phenotypic adaptation under enriched conditions. Now, here's what makes Hart Island remarkable. The soil there wasn't enriched. No compounds were added, and no amendments were introduced. The only variable was the reintroduction of human remains, some long decayed, while others were only recently interred. Somehow, those remains have triggered an event in the soil."

She glances at the group before continuing, as if translating her own findings. "In simpler terms, the plants are changing their behavior as if they've detected something new in their environment, something they recognize as once alive."

Meera lets that sink in before continuing. "Additionally, soil microbial sequencing indicates a sustained elevation of certain symbiotic bacterial strains, correlating with the highest legacy signal concentration zones. Silent echoes of past life, a kind of activation or relay. Whatever is happening beneath Hart Island, it's not residual. It's interactive."

Theo raises an eyebrow, prompting her to add, "That means the microbes aren't just breaking things down, they're responding, reorganizing, and possibly forming new partnerships with the roots above them. The system is behaving more like a conversation."

Meera continues, "We're also tracking trace elemental migration patterns. Zinc mostly, with manganese and boron. It's likely pulled or pushed by biological activity rather than abiotic leaching. We may witness a biochemical echo of human presence if these correlations hold.

A kind of terrestrial inheritance network carried and reshaped by plant-microbe interactions."

She softens her tone. "In plain terms, it's as if elements that once circulated in us—trace metals, nutrients—are now being carried forward through the living system. Recycled and reorganized with purpose."

Camila nods into her camera, adding, "These changes are all consistent with what we observed in Normandy. The plants appear to be reacting to microbial shifts in the soil, subtle but persistent. This reinforces what we've said from the beginning. Legacy influence isn't limited to microbial inheritance or soil-bound signatures. It's ecological."

She gestures toward the screen. "What we're seeing suggests that when human material reenters the environment, it becomes part of a larger biological feedback loop. Life remembered in structure."

Theo breaks the silent contemplation that follows as everyone simultaneously stares off into the distance. "How is this even possible? If there was no enrichment, no catalyst introduced, then what changed? What's doing the work?"

Camila straightens, already pulling up a slide deck of her own. "That's what we've been trying to understand. My team has been running parallel simulations using archived soil samples from both Hart Island and Normandy. In both cases, the microbial communities respond in ways that appear anticipatory. It's as if they're engaging in a form of chemical communication. We think quorum-sensing activity may be at play, triggered by residual proteins from human remains. Even in highly decayed material, those proteins may still act as an ignition."

She pauses, then continues more cautiously. "We also can't ignore the possibility that the soil itself retains a kind of informational momentum. A reactive imprint that influences microbial organization. The patterns are hard to dismiss, even at this early stage."

Seeing the uncertainty in their faces, she adds quietly, "If that sounds abstract, think of the soil more like a living memory than a medium. Once touched by life, it keeps some trace of how to organize itself around it."

Theo exhales slowly, absorbing the implications.

Camila jumps back in before the silence can stretch too far. "One more detail. There's been a marked increase in fungal load across the test sites. We're seeing robust mycelial growth, particularly around the same root zones where gene expression is shifting. A mycelial network may form, bridging plant roots like a subterranean web. These fungal pathways might facilitate the transmission of biochemical cues, maybe even genetic fragments, between plants. We've underestimated how much communication might be happening belowground."

She clicks to a new slide. "There's something else. Researchers noticed an unfamiliar fragrance above the soil. It's subtle. Not floral. Not putrid. Something noticeable. The soil appeared somewhat aerated as decomposition occurred, as if gas exchange had increased through microbial or fungal tunneling. This aeration may enhance the transmission of volatile compounds or chemical signals."

Julia leans into her camera with a bewildered laugh. "Wait. Are you telling me the Earth passed gas, and that's helping to transmit the genetic information?"

Theo raises his eyebrows, half-grinning as he lifts a hand in mock surrender. "King of the lab. I did not see that coming."

Julia smirks and narrows her eyes at her screen. "Theo."

Camila smiles, unshaken. "Crude, but fairly accurate. That fragrance might be part of the signal rather than a byproduct."

She glances around the screen. "It's multiple organisms reacting in an ecological chorus."

Meera picks up the thread. "All of these realizations—altered gene expression, microbial shifts, fungal networks, even the gaseous transmissions—will need to be continually observed and tested at each of our coalition sites. Where experiments or replications are underway, we need coordinated protocols to track expected and emergent changes. This is no longer about single findings. It's about patterns that might point to something far more systemic."

She pauses just long enough to signal a shift. "Sonia, can you give us a quick media update? What do you see between coverage trends, public feedback, and where the messaging might need reinforcement?"

Sonia states with a measured tone. "The volume hasn't slowed. If anything, it's getting louder. We're tracking coverage across every continent now. Most of it is neutral or cautiously supportive, but there's a noticeable uptick in sensationalist framing."

She taps a few keys, and a small heat map of media activity appears on-screen. "Right now, Europe and Latin America are showing the most sustained engagement, especially around the ethics of soil sampling. Religious groups are weighing in. Some raise alarms about sacred ground desecration, while others are curious, seeing this as evidence of soul resonance or spiritual continuity."

Sonia glances at the team. "In the U.S., though, we've hit a split. Mainstream outlets are holding the line with factual reporting, but fringe sites are starting to paint this as either a miracle or a government cover-up. Dell Children's communications team is monitoring the trend and preparing a joint op-ed to recenter the narrative around education, research transparency, and the medical possibilities. Moreover, we'll need faces to represent the data. That's where Camila's and Dr. Kamara's public appearances have been so effective. We should consider doing more of that. Share small, personal stories from each site."

She finishes with a steady breath. "There's momentum, but there's risk too. People want answers. If we don't give them the real story, then someone else will."

She pauses, then adds, "One more thing. The Shepherd's Stand Alliance hasn't gone quiet. Despite Senator Greer's statement, they're pushing the idea that our fieldwork could 'reactivate' or contaminate old burial zones. It's misinformation rooted in misunderstanding, but it's spreading fast enough that we're tracking and correcting it."

She glances at another window open on her screen. "Later this week, Andrew and I have a meeting scheduled with the hospital's media team to discuss a more formal press conference. We're considering a moderated format. Something that allows for direct engagement. Rather than issuing another static statement, we'll field questions in a structured setting. If we do this right, it could cut through the noise and restore a bit of balance to the public conversation."

Meera nods and checks the time. "Let's hold it here for today. At the same time next week, come prepared with any new findings, especially replication data and site comparisons. We'll regroup and build from there."

The screens begin to go dark one by one. Some wave, others simply disconnect. The meeting ends with a collective breath, a quiet moment stretching across continents.

Later in the week, back at home, Sonia sits on the edge of the couch with her laptop open and notecards spread across the coffee table. She's dressed in a blouse that looks both professional and camera-ready, testing different ways to phrase her opening remarks. Andrew stands in the kitchen stirring a pot, glancing over with quiet encouragement.

Junie is curled up in the armchair nearby, holding a stack of flashcards she put together with Dad's help. "Okay, Mommy," she grins. Next question. What if someone asks whether you believe the soil can think?"

Sonia stifles a laugh, setting her laptop aside. "I'd say that soil doesn't think. But it does respond. Just like our skin responds to sunlight or our bodies to heat. The reactions aren't conscious."

Junie raises another card dramatically. "What if someone says this is all just a hoax to get funding?"

Sonia tilts her head. "Then I'll tell them our funding hasn't even caught up with the questions we're being asked to answer. We're doing this because the evidence is real, and frankly, too big to ignore."

Junie hesitates before reading the next card. "Okay... kind of a gross one." She swallows. "How does the soil use the bodies? What does it do with them?"

She looks uneasy, then adds, "This was Dad's question."

Sonia blinks, clearly taken with the question. "That's a brilliant question. The soil breaks them down, sure, but it also distributes what's left. Nutrients, organic compounds, proteins, and fragments of DNA. Those get taken up by microbes, fungi, and maybe even plants. It's not used in the way we think of tools. It's more like absorption and translation."

Junie flips to another card. "So then, what does it mean to walk and breathe over that same soil? Does that make us part of it? Can I still walk barefoot on the grass?"

Sonia gazes at her daughter and smiles gently. "In a way, yes. We're always part of it. The air we breathe and the food we eat are all filtered through the same ground. So, maybe we're not separate from it at all. Maybe we're just the next layer. To answer your last question, yes, you can still walk barefoot through the grass. That's one way we remain connected to the land and the life beneath it. Walking barefoot simply means you're part of the conversation."

Andrew walks over with two mugs of tea, handing one to Sonia and resting a hand briefly on her shoulder. "She's tougher than the moderator already."

Junie beams. "Obviously. I made the hard questions."

The three of them have spent weeks like this, folding Junie into conversations that once lived only in labs and meeting rooms. It's slower, more patient work. Pausing to explain and to listen, but they've come to realize it matters. These talks won't end tonight; they're shaping the way she'll see the world.

The following morning, Sonia and Andrew stand in the wings of the Hogg Memorial Auditorium on the University of Texas campus. The historic venue hums with anticipation, with its warm wooden paneling and long, curved rows of orange theater seats. Built in the 1930s, the space carries the gravity of generations. Governors, poets, and scientists have all addressed the people of Austin beneath the heavy velvet curtain.

Outside, the thick shade of sprawling live oaks offers a welcome break from the summer heat of the Texas sun. Inside, quiet tension hangs in the air as sound techs do their final checks and students with clipboards adjust camera angles for the live stream. A podium stands center stage, flanked by two upholstered chairs for the moderator and guest expert.

Sonia sits beside Andrew, both framed in the muted glow of the studio lights. She smooths the front of her charcoal-gray jacket and checks her reflection in the tablet's dark glass. Her ivory blouse was chosen for neutrality on camera, neither blue nor green to distort the overlays. A small silver pin near her collar catches the light.

Andrew, meanwhile, reviews the opening notes on his tablet, his jacket a simple navy that grounds the pair visually—her precision softened by his understated calm. The overall impression is one of practiced partnership: two people aligned in purpose, each steadying the other before the broadcast begins.

Sonia glances down at her notecards one last time. The lights above dim slightly. A stagehand gives the cue.

It's time.

The moderator steps forward, a professor from the university's school of journalism, familiar to many in the audience. She welcomes the attendees and introduces the format as a live, moderated conversation followed by questions submitted in advance and screened for clarity and tone.

"Today's discussion," she says, "is about the science we've been reading about as well as the greater story behind the science. The story of how we choose to participate in the health of our planet, how we honor our ancestors, and how our ancestors and the earth might be whispering back to future generations."

She gestures to the guests seated at center stage. "Please welcome Dr. Andrew Turbin and Mrs. Sonia Turbin, whose work with the international coalition has guided much of what we'll be discussing today."

The audience applauds sincerely. Andrew nods with a small smile; Sonia offers a gracious wave.

"Thank you," Sonia begins. "It's easy to forget that the real world keeps moving while we're buried in lab reports and sequencing data. People are listening and wondering about what we're finding and what it means. We're here to share what we know and to be honest about what we don't."

Andrew adds, "And hopefully, to explain the science in a way that connects with what matters most to all of us, how we live with the land, not apart from it."

Sonia nods. "Because the ground beneath us is more than a container. It's active. It's reactive. And in some ways, it might even be communicative. That's where our work begins."

There's a brief, intentional pause.

The moderator nods appreciatively and offers her first question. "Dr. Turbin, let's start with that word, 'communicative.' Would you explain what that means in a scientific context, and how that idea fits with what the coalition has uncovered so far?"

Andrew looks at the audience, clasping his hands. "In science, we use the word 'communication' to describe how systems exchange information through signals. Chemical, electrical, and molecular. When we talk about the soil being communicative, we're describing a living network of exchange. Plants adjust their gene expression, microbes shift their populations, and fungi build bridges across root systems. Those aren't random events. They're coordinated responses. Something changes in one area of the soil, and another area reacts. The deeper we look, the more it appears that information and material are being transferred."

He glances toward Sonia before continuing. "It's still early, but the evidence suggests these interactions may be fundamental to how ecosystems regulate themselves after disturbance or decay."

Sonia continues, "And that perspective opens a larger question about what role we play in that network, especially when our remains return to it."

The moderator nods appreciatively, then pivots. "That leads me to something a lot of people are asking. You've talked about communication and memory, but how are we expected to believe that burying someone without a sealed container could actually lead to better health? To benefit? Isn't that the opposite of what we've always been taught about hygiene and contamination? More than that, what of our respect for the dead?"

Sonia acknowledges the question first. "That's a fair concern, and one we both shared when this research began." She looks to Andrew.

Andrew picks up smoothly. "Historically, sealed burial practices evolved to protect public health from cholera, plague, and poor sanitation. Those were real threats, and some still are. But it's also true that most pathogens, including respiratory viruses like SARS-CoV-2, lose viability quickly after death. Once circulation and temperature control end, the biological environment shifts, and viruses can't replicate. What remains is organic material. Cells, proteins, and trace elements that the soil's microbial network can safely break down."

He pauses, then continues. "Under controlled, natural conditions, the soil doesn't just absorb what's left behind; it reorganizes it. The microbial communities adapt and stabilize. We monitor these sites for contaminants, and when proper time and temperature thresholds are observed,

THE LIVING SYSTEM

the risk of infection falls below measurable levels. What we're seeing isn't uncontrolled decay or contamination. What we're seeing is reintegration."

He gestures lightly with one hand. "At Hart Island, for example, we didn't add anything artificial or enrich the soil. We simply allowed natural contact between organic matter and the living substrate. Even so, we observed microbial and fungal shifts and corresponding gene-expression changes in nearby plant life. These aren't sterile fields; they're living systems showing adaptive, restorative behavior. It's about understanding balance with nature."

Sonia nods. "We're still in the early stages, but what's becoming clear is that nature knows how to process what we leave behind. Possibly better than we do when we seal it in metal and concrete."

The moderator probes into the question a little deeper. "You've both spoken about what happens biologically, but what's the larger goal here? Why pursue this line of research? What are you hoping to accomplish?"

Andrew exchanges a glance with Sonia before answering. "At its core, the goal is restoration. We want to understand how human material—our nutrients and chemistry—can return safely and beneficially to the environment. If we can map those processes, we can design burial and memorial systems that heal rather than isolate. Systems that restore soil vitality, carbon balance, and biodiversity instead of locking potential away in sealed containers."

Sonia adds, "And beyond the science, it's also about redefining our relationship with death and the earth itself. We've built walls—metaphorical and literal—between ourselves and the natural cycles that sustain us. What we're doing isn't dismantling tradition; it's exploring how reverence and renewal can coexist."

Andrew nods. "The end goal is resilience. Healthier soil means healthier ecosystems. And healthier ecosystems, in turn, support human life. It's all connected. We're trying to change what happens after grief, so that life continues to benefit from the lives that came before."

The moderator listens closely before continuing. "There's been some talk about these so-called 'Legacy Gardens' as test sites in other countries experimenting with new burial approaches. Would you tell us what that looks like? What are you proposing, exactly? Are we talking about burying the dead in public parks?"

Andrew smiles faintly at the phrasing. "Not quite. Legacy Gardens are purpose-built research and memorial spaces. Each one operates under strict environmental and ethical oversight. They're designed to study soil vitality, carbon storage, biodiversity, and air quality while maintaining boundaries and pathogen controls."

Sonia adds, "They're also places of remembrance. They're spaces that invite reflection and renewal. In dense cities, we can't expand cemeteries endlessly, but we can create environments that sustain both people and the planet. We need burial options that are sustainable, safe, and community-centered. These gardens can serve multiple roles, including mourning, regeneration, and scientific observation. It's a practical application."

Andrew continues, "Right now, these gardens are fenced and managed like any other ecological or memorial site. However, in the future, we may see more integrated designs."

The moderator pulls out a printed page. "This next one is from social media. While it's phrased a little dramatically, it reflects a real undercurrent of public anxiety." She clears her throat and reads. "If the earth is absorbing our DNA, and plants are 'remembering' the dead, are we on the edge of resurrecting something we shouldn't? Is this science or summoning?"

She glances over the rim of her glasses at both of them. "It's a serious question, even if the tone is speculative. There's fear wrapped up in this idea that something unnatural is taking root."

Andrew and Sonia look at one another. It's clear that Andrew is ready to lead their answer. "I'm glad this question made it through the screeners, because we need to talk about fear. What's happening isn't resurrection. It's a reorganization. The DNA fragments we detect in soil aren't rebuilding people. They're being broken down and redistributed by complex ecosystems, forming part of the nutrient and microbial cycles that sustain new growth."

Sonia adds, "And that's what's beautiful about it. We've always returned to the earth. What's new is our ability to observe it and recognize that the process is more structured and more reactive than we previously understood."

The moderator takes a measured breath and lifts another card, printed on thicker paper, visibly folded from being carried around. "This question came from a clergy member in Kansas. It reads, 'What you're describing may be natural, but is it reverent? Have we forgotten what it means to care for the dead, to hold them with dignity and spiritual intention? We're not compost. We're sacred.'"

She turns to them both. "How do you respond to that?"

Sonia's expression softens. "I hear that, and I don't take it lightly. Reverence is about what we choose to honor, even in decay. For centuries, different cultures have found sacred meaning in very different burial practices. Fire. Water. Earth. None of those rituals lose dignity because the body changes form."

Andrew adds quietly, "We treat every research site as both laboratory and memorial. Each one is monitored, documented, and protected. We don't see data points. We see lives, and the systems that hold them."

Sonia continues, "We're not asking people to surrender their traditions. We're asking them to see death as part of transformation, and transformation as something worthy of hushed respect." Her gaze moves gently across the audience. "For some, that might mean prayer. For others, a silent pause. For us, as researchers, it means ensuring that every test site is treated as more than a dataset. It's a memorial."

The moderator seems lost in thought and then turns to the next card. "This question comes from a health policy researcher in Toronto. It reads, 'Has the coalition discussed a tiered community opt-in system? Something that allows regions to participate based on cultural alignment, health infrastructure, and informed consent rather than a one-size-fits-all approach?'"

Andrew nods appreciatively. "That's a vital question, and one that's being handled primarily by regional health and environmental agencies. Our coalition's role is to provide the data and field observations that help those agencies make informed decisions. We don't set policy; we inform it."

He glances toward Sonia, who continues, "What we are doing is making sure our research is transparent and accessible, so that communities and policymakers have the evidence they need to decide what participation should look like in their own regions. Each culture, each governing body will determine what's appropriate based on values, resources, and readiness."

Andrew adds, "In that sense, it's already a kind of tiered system. Some areas are observing, others are piloting. That flexibility is important, but it's guided by public policy and community consent, not by us as scientists."

Sonia pauses and then continues more personally. "This isn't about imposing an agenda. It's about creating space for participation at different levels and in distinctive ways, participating without fear or pressure. Consent isn't a checkbox. It's a dialogue, and that dialogue will look different everywhere."

The moderator sets the card down, looks up, and pauses a moment. "One last question. It's a personal one, but it's already been mentioned in some of the background articles and public records. Both of your families have multi-generation crypts, places where your parents, grandparents, and extended relatives are honored? That kind of lineage represents a long tradition of memorial care. Given all that you've shared today, what do you plan to do personally? Will you be setting the example?"

Sonia draws in a quiet breath. Her hands rest in her lap, fingers tighten slightly. She was expecting this question, had rehearsed it in her mind, but now that it's here, her voice wavers at the edge of emotion.

"Yes," she says while looking at Andrew. "We do have family crypts. In fact, both sides of our families have long histories of memorials. These are places we visit on holidays and anniversaries. Those places matter. They still matter."

She pauses to collect herself, blinking once to steady the moisture rising in her eyes. Looking out into the audience, she continues. "This wasn't an easy decision. Andrew and I talked about it at length. We brought it to our family. We asked hard questions. We had late-night debates, and more than one moment of silence, when the weight of legacy felt like too much to speak against."

Sonia stops as she looks down, placing a hand on her chest. Andrew continues without hesitation. "Eventually, we came to a shared conclusion that the best way to honor our ancestors is to consider what they've taught us about responsibility and giving back. For us, that means participating fully in this moment."

A hush settles over the auditorium.

Andrew and Sonia look at one another as Sonia continues, "We've agreed to participate in Austin's first Legacy Garden. When the time comes, our family remains will go there. In dialogue and agreement with our families, we're choosing to become part of the living system, reverently and publicly."

CHAPTER 24
CLOSER TO HOME

The house feels quieter than it should. The lights are softer, the air still. Sonia steps out of her heels at the door, leaving them neatly beside the bench where Junie's sneakers are already kicked half-underneath. Andrew walks up behind her and catches her gaze with a look that expresses a mix of pride, relief, and a touch of awe. He doesn't say anything at first. He just pulls her into a long hug, gently resting his chin on her shoulder.

Junie peeks around the corner, her hair a bit mussed from her nap in the car. "Mommy, you didn't cry. I thought you might."

Sonia smiles as she steps back from Andrew. "I almost did, but then I remembered your flashcards."

Junie beams, holding up her notebook like a badge. "I told you they'd help."

They settle into the living room together with Sonia in her usual corner of the couch, Andrew in the armchair with his legs pulled up, and Junie nestled between them on the rug with her sketchbook.

Andrew breaks the quiet first. "You know, you were great. You guided the whole conversation. I watched that room shift with you."

Sonia exhales, still holding some of the tension in her shoulders. "I'm grateful for your participation. It sure didn't feel like I was guiding them.

It felt more like I let it become real. People want to believe in something, but they also want to be heard."

Junie flips her sketchbook toward them, displaying a rough drawing of the stage, complete with two caricatures and a little heart hovering between. "That's you and Dad. I gave you superhero capes."

Sonia leans forward to kiss her forehead. "You're the real hero. I only got through it because of you."

Andrew nods. "And now we're on the record. Austin's first Legacy Garden. That's not a small step."

Sonia looks between them, quiet for a moment. "It's not just about setting an example. It's about making room for what comes next. I don't want Junie to grow up afraid of it. I want her to understand that we're all part of something bigger, even after."

Junie glances up. "Does that mean I get to design your gardens?"

Sonia laughs. "Not yet, but maybe you'll help us plant something there. Something that grows."

Andrew shifts, his tone turning practical. "You know what's next," he says, glancing at Sonia. "We need to start planning for the move. Once we get the green light, it's time to bring them home."

Sonia nods slowly, her expression calm and reflective. "We said we would, and everyone gave us their blessing to bring the ancestors to Austin. I still can't believe how willing everyone was in the end."

"We did the hard part already," Andrew says. "The conversations and the permissions. It's all lined up. Now it's logistics. Timelines. Coordination with the cemeteries."

"And care," Sonia adds. "We need to do this with care. It's family."

The next morning, Dell Children's Medical Center feels unusually quiet. The atrium lights are dimmed just enough to soften the hum of early routines. Theo rests against a column near the entrance, sipping from a takeaway cup with his badge still clipped to the outside of his jacket. Andrew stands beside him, hands in his pockets, eyes tracking the elevators.

They don't have to wait long. Meera steps out of the elevator with her shoulder bag already slung and her scarf knotted neatly at her collar. She smiles when she sees them, with a quiet weight to her expression. She has the kind of calm that only comes after decisions are final.

Theo straightens. "You're really going, huh?"

Meera nods, shifting her bag. "For now. My dean recalled me. We always knew my time in Austin was limited. It was just a question of when. The site in India is nearly ready, and with local permissions in place, I need to be there in person. It's time to stop watching from here."

Andrew offers a wry smile. "We knew this day was coming. Doesn't mean we like it."

Meera laughs softly. "I'll miss the company, but I won't miss the chai. American chai is so bland."

Theo grins, clearly pleased with her jab. "Especially the company and the wit."

She reaches out and squeezes both their arms. "This isn't goodbye. It's just the next part. We'll be in touch. Weekly calls. Data drops. Probably more WhatsApp messages than you want."

Andrew's voice softens. "It won't be the same without you in the lab."

Meera looks at him, then Theo. "It's not supposed to be. That means it mattered."

She turns, and the three of them begin the slow walk down the hall toward the main exit. As they round the corner past the genetics wing, the hallway comes into view, lined on both sides with lab staff. Some wear scrubs, others still have goggles perched on their heads or gloves in their back pockets. There are nods, small waves, and a few tight smiles that don't quite hide the emotion behind them.

A few clap quietly as Meera passes, and someone near the end of the line hands her a folded note with a single marigold tucked into the crease. Meera takes it with a grateful nod, her throat tight.

Theo murmurs, "You've got a fan club."

Andrew adds, "They wanted to be here. All of them."

Meera swallows and offers a small bow of her head as she walks. "I don't know what to say."

"You already did," Theo replies. "Over and over again."

As soon as the doors close behind her, Theo and Andrew exchange glances and then break into a light jog down the corridor.

"The coalition call starts in three," Andrew says.

"Two, if they're early," Theo mutters, clutching his coffee like a lifeline.

They duck into the lab just as the screen flickers to life. Faces begin populating the call from Japan, Brazil, the Netherlands, and others across the U.S.

Theo slides into his chair and unmutes with a practiced swipe. "Good morning, good afternoon, good evening, wherever you're dialing in from. You've got Theo and Andrew here in Austin. Meera's on her way back to India, so she'll miss today's session, but we'll catch her up on the rerun."

He gives the camera a nod. "Camila, let's start with you. You were beginning to outline progress in São Paulo last time we met. Can you update us on the Legacy Garden development there?"

Camila's square lights up as she unmutes, sunlight slanting in from the window behind her. A map is pinned behind her on the wall, with color-coded markings clustered along the city's eastern edge.

"We've secured three candidate sites," she begins, her voice crisp. "All are within reach of existing infrastructure but buffered enough to maintain ecological separation. Soil tests came back positive for microbial diversity and drainage. We've started phase-one conditioning with low-impact compost to see how the base profile responds."

She pauses to swipe to another screen. "We're also in formal talks with São Paulo's public health department. They've expressed support in principle, pending results from our six-month viability review. Additionally, we're planning listening sessions with local community leaders next week, trying to keep this as collaborative as possible from the ground up."

As she wraps, Theo scrolls through the screen. "Thanks, Camila. Let's open it up. Anyone else who's begun local outreach, pilot planning, or community engagement? What's up on your end?"

A voice from Tokyo picks up next. Dr. Saito bows his head slightly before speaking. "We've partnered with a university cemetery. One that's historically significant but underused. The city council granted preliminary approval to transform a small portion into a monitored ecological test site. Local schools have shown interest in contributing to soil readings and documentation as a science-education initiative."

Then comes Dr. Helena van Dijk from the Netherlands. "We're

pursuing a retrofit model," she explains. "Rather than carving new spaces, we're evaluating how existing rural cemeteries might accommodate regenerative practices. A team is compiling data on soil permeability and microbe populations."

She hesitates before continuing. "That said, one of our control sites has yielded almost no biological response. The microbial counts have declined instead of stabilizing, and pH levels are drifting upward, suggesting we may have over-conditioned or introduced an imbalance."

Theo looks up from his screen. "Is it local contamination? Agricultural runoff?"

"Possibly," Helena replies. "There's a dairy operation less than a kilometer away. We're testing groundwater to rule out external influence, but for now, it's an anomaly."

A short silence follows before Dr. Kwame Mensah from Ghana chimes in, his tone calm and grounding. "Our conversations with tribal elders have been careful and respectful. While urban municipalities are curious, the emphasis has been on preserving ritual integrity. We may see pilot testing in smaller villages that are willing to explore hybrid ceremonial-scientific burials. It's slow yet sacred."

Lastly, Dr. Élodie Garnier in France gives a concise but promising update. "While we're still watching Hart Island, we've also received conditional clearance to begin a secondary pilot outside Montpellier. This site will run in tandem with our comparative microbial studies. We're particularly focused on seasonal variation and gene exchange at the root level."

Andrew leans forward slightly as Élodie finishes. "I'll jump in with one more," he says. "We've re-tested the Normandy site, focusing specifically on four control plots that should, by all accounts, show nothing. No exposure, no known burials, and no site enrichment."

He taps on his tablet and pulls up a shared screen. "These plots were selected for their distance from all mapped gravesites, over two hundred meters in most cases. The soil history shows no recorded disturbance, and there's no vegetation pattern that would suggest prior anomalies."

He looks up. "Surprisingly, we're detecting activity. It's relatively mild and has a narrow band, but it's consistent enough to register in the microbial and RNA expression scans. The same two markers first appeared in the enriched zones six months ago. We've already double-checked the equipment. Re-ran the assays. Still there."

Theo raises an eyebrow. "So, Helena's site is quiet, but yours is alive when it shouldn't be."

Andrew nods. "Exactly. Opposite ends of the spectrum. Which means we're probably missing something in our model. Perhaps there's some environmental trigger we haven't accounted for."

Sonia, off camera, murmurs, "Or something the model can't see yet."

The call goes silent briefly.

Theo exhales. "Alright. Let's document both anomalies and flag them for cross-review. It's good to have something that doesn't fit. It's how we'll know where to look next."

A few faces on the call shift forward, visibly intrigued.

Andrew continues, "Overall, results are consistent, and this appears to confirm questions about proximity influence and whether legacy signals might persist in nearby soil, even if not directly used." He glances at the screen, gauging the reactions. "It's subtle. The signal mirrors what we saw early in São Paulo and Normandy's initial zone. If the soil can 'remember' from a distance and carry influence across untouched boundaries, then it redefines how we think about environmental inheritance. It becomes a question of what's adjacent rather than what's buried."

The coalition gradually draws to a close for the day, while several hours later, on the other side of the planet, Meera steps off a narrow train platform just outside Hyderabad. The morning air is warm and touched with dust. A driver in a white cap lifts a hand from beside an aging Land Rover, and she waves back, adjusting the strap of her bag and making her way across the uneven pavement.

The road to the burial site takes them past fields of marigolds and turmeric, then narrows as they wind into a grove of teak and neem. Somewhere along the way, Meera dozes off with her head resting against the window, lulled by the motion and the warmth. The nap takes her by surprise. When she stirs awake, the driver is slowing near a clearing, and her neck aches from the angle.

She stretches slightly and rubs her eyes, blinking at the sudden light outside. "That flight is no joke," she mutters, mostly to herself. "Austin to

Delhi and then a train to here. It's like chasing time backwards and sideways."

When the vehicle finally stops, she steps out into a sun-dappled clearing marked by a rusted gate and a simple sign in Marathi and English. Beyond it, the land opens into soft, furrowed earth surrounded by native trees, quiet and expectant. A breeze carries the smell of the soil and something much older: memory.

Meera pauses at the threshold. This isn't just any site. She grew up near Pune, just a few hours from here. Childhood weekends spent with cousins in the hills, school trips to nearby temples, the rhythm of language, monsoon, and market noise all return in fragments. She'd never imagined this region would become one of the keystones in their global study, but now it feels inevitable. Fated.

She walks the perimeter slowly, passing low stone markers and half-covered mounds where recent soil studies have been flagged. Nearby, a group of local schoolchildren is helping clear the underbrush under the supervision of an older man in a saffron kurta. He's one of the community elders who signed the land use agreement.

Meera breathes in deeply. The air is alive with the scent of earth, leaf oil, and the faint bitterness of wood smoke. She kneels near a newly demarcated boundary and presses her fingers into the soil.

"This is where it begins," she murmurs. "Again."

The elder in the saffron kurta approaches slowly, nodding with familiarity. "Dr. Rao," he says graciously. "I am Ravi Deshmukh. We've spoken by phone, yes?"

She rises to her feet and returns the nod. "Yes, thank you for meeting me here."

Ravi gestures toward the open plot. "You have access to the entire northern quadrant for sampling and observation. Burial preparations are restricted to the central and eastern lots until we receive further clearance. No heavy machinery is allowed on the inner perimeter. The school has granted temporary use of their solar-powered monitoring equipment."

He offers a paper folder. "All permits are in here, with signatures from the council and cultural board. If any questions arise, call me directly. We want this done with transparency and honor."

Meera takes the folder gently, her gratitude quiet but deep. "It will be."

She tucks the folder under her arm and says, "I grew up in Shendurwadi. Not far from here. Childhood mornings walking to school beneath banyan trees, evenings spent on terraces with my grandfather sharing stories. This region shaped how I see the world. I arrived early to spend a little time with the land before the work begins. As someone who belongs to this place, it's important to me to reconnect first. I need the soil to recognize me before I ask anything of it."

Ravi nods with a deeper respect now. "Then you understand what's at stake. It is good you came with more than data."

He gestures toward a stone bench shaded by a neem tree, and they walk slowly toward it. "We have not touched this land for over a generation," he says. "There are old stories tied to it. Some are cautionary while others are hopeful. No one has planted here since the river changed course. It's been waiting."

Meera sits gently, resting the folder on her lap. "Waiting for what?"

"For purpose," Ravi says simply. "For someone who remembers how to listen. Most people come only to extract. When you speak of recognition and memory, however, it tells me you know this is more than a site. It's a witness."

She looks out across the field, letting his words settle. "We'll begin with small introductions," she says. "Soil cores, microbial sequencing. Observation before disturbance."

He smiles. "That is the right order."

A bird calls from the grove's edge, and the wind shifts, lifting a curl of dust down the path. Meera exhales slowly, as if syncing her breath with the rhythm of the place.

"I've never done fieldwork this close to home," she says softly.

Ravi glances at her. "That is a blessing and a burden. The two will guide your hand."

Later that afternoon, Meera quietly leaves the grove and drives to Shendurwadi. The road climbs through terraced hills and quiet mango orchards, the colors shifting from amber dust to deep greens as the elevation rises. The driver drops her at the edge of a footpath, and she walks the rest of the way alone.

The tree is still there. It's massive and regal. A wild neem with gnarled limbs that stretch out in every direction. Her grandmother had asked to be buried here, directly in the soil, wrapped only in cotton. Meera approaches slowly and lowers herself to the earth at the base of the trunk.

She doesn't speak at first. She just breathes and lets her hands settle onto the ground. The bark is cool against her back. After a long silence, she begins.

"I've come back to listen. We're asking the world to hear what lives beneath us, and I can't do that unless I first hear you. Not the memory of you. You. In this place. In this soil."

A small wind rustles the leaves overhead.

"I don't know what we're going to find. But I promise we're honoring the moment. We'll disturb as little as possible. We'll record everything we can. I'll carry what you taught me into every lab, every call, every choice."

She places her palm flat on the ground with her eyes closed. "Thank you for making me brave."

It is now about 6:30 a.m. in Austin, and Theo stands in front of his bathroom mirror, half-dressed, toothbrush in hand. His tie is still draped over the towel hook, and the news plays softly from the other room without sound. Sunlight cuts through the kitchen blinds like gold dust, catching on the edge of a family photo frame left on the counter.

He finishes brushing, rinses, and then moves to the photo. It's an older image of his father, laughing at the edge of a fishing boat, baseball cap backwards and eyes squinting against the light. Eight years gone now. Cancer.

Theo presses his thumb gently against the glass. "Morning, Dad." His voice is just above a whisper. "I know you'd say this is all a little out there, but you'd also be the first to ask me to explain it over beer."

He pauses, eyes still on the photo. "You always said, 'Wouldn't it be great if you were presented with an opportunity to commune with the spirits? If it happened right here and now, and you could open up to it?'"

Theo's voice softens even more. "That moment is happening now, Dad. And we're opening up to it."

He exhales, heavier than he means to. "We're getting closer to something that makes sense. Something we can test, repeat, and prove. I don't know what you'd think of Legacy Gardens or microbial sequencing, but I hope you'd see that we're asking the right questions. That we're trying to understand how the living system carries us forward."

Theo looks up at the ceiling. "If you're watching, maybe nudge our results this week. I could use a little statistical favor."

He chuckles softly, ties the knot around his collar, and grabs his keys.

He drives through familiar streets just beginning to stir with dog walkers, joggers, and the first few kids heading to school. His destination is a quiet café between a yoga studio and a dry cleaner, a place his mother claimed to be "the only place in town that understands a real breakfast."

She's already seated when he arrives, reading a folded newspaper with her coffee untouched. Her posture, as always, is regal without being rigid. She's stoic and composed in a linen blouse and pearl studs. She was June Cleaver with a Texan spine to Theo's childhood friends. Unshakable. Not fussy. Full of grace under pressure.

"You're ten minutes early," she says, folding the paper without looking up.

"Which means I'm five minutes late by your standards," he replies, and leans down to kiss her cheek.

She lifts her eyes to his for a moment, long enough to say, without words, that she sees him. That she knows something is shifting.

"You've been working too much," she says.

"It's not just work, Mom. We're on the edge of something big. Big enough that I almost skipped breakfast, but then I remembered how you interrogate empty chairs."

She doesn't even blink.

Theo chuckles and shakes his head. "Tough room."

She stirs her coffee gently, the spoon barely making a sound. "I figured as much. You've got that look your father used to get. Like something's talking to you, and you're just trying to figure out if you're brave enough to answer."

Theo shifts in his seat, reaching for his water glass more for something to do than out of thirst. He swirls it once and sets it back down.

"Well, maybe he's sending backup," he says, trying for a smile that doesn't quite land.

His mother doesn't respond right away. She folds her napkin in her lap, calm and unreadable. The silence stretches just long enough to feel intentional.

Theo clears his throat. "Okay. No backup. Got it."

He lets the quiet settle for a breath longer, resting his elbows on the table. "We're learning something about death, Mom. Not in a morbid way. In a practical, living-soil kind of way. The way roots grow through memory, and how the earth holds more than we've understood. It's like it doesn't just absorb our remains. It translates it. Makes something new out of it."

She raises an eyebrow, listening without interrupting.

He presses on. "It's not hocus-pocus. We've got RNA shifts, microbial shifts, and plants reacting to what's below. It's science, but it feels like a kind of ceremonial respect. Like the ground knows something about who we were. If that's true, then maybe we owe it more respect than just concrete vaults and chemical embalming."

His mother sets her coffee down. "You're saying death teaches us how to live."

Theo nods. "Or at least how to keep listening after someone's gone."

She studies him for a long moment. "Listening is good," she says finally. "Most people spend half their lives talking past what's right in front of them."

Theo exhales through his nose, a quiet laugh. "You used to say that when Dad and I argued about homework."

"I said it because you both liked to be right," she replies, a faint smile forming. "But being right isn't the same as being present. You can't learn anything if you're too busy defending what you already know."

He nods, tracing a small circle on the table with his thumb. "That's what the research feels like sometimes. Like we're defending the way we've always done things instead of asking what the world's been trying to show us."

She lifts her cup again, her voice firm. "Then stop defending. Listen harder. The ground's not the only thing that remembers."

Theo looks up, caught by the weight of that line. "You mean you?"

"I mean all of us," she says. "Family, places, the things we leave unsaid. You think you're discovering something new, but maybe you're just learning the language we forgot."

He sits back, the words landing deeper than he expects. "You make it sound simple."

"It's not simple," she says, setting her cup down again. "It's work. But you've always been good at that."

A small silence settles between them, lighter than before. Outside, the street is beginning to hum with traffic.

Theo glances toward the window. "You should come see the site sometime. The soil samples alone would convert you."

She chuckles softly. "Let's start with breakfast. One discovery at a time."

Theo smiles, a real one this time. "Fair enough."

She adjusts her napkin and begins buttering her toast with steady precision. "Just promise me one thing," she says without looking up.

"What's that?"

"When you listen to the ground," she says, "make sure you still hear the living."

Theo watches her for a moment, then nods. "I will."

CHAPTER 25
THE FUTURE, AS PROMISED

Ten years later, Austin's Performing Arts Center glows in the early summer light. The concrete façade is softened by clusters of parents, siblings, and friends gathering along the shaded breezeways and entry steps. Banners ripple slightly in the breeze, and rows of folding chairs line the open plaza in front of the stage entrance. The marquee reads in bold digital type: Alpha High School Commencement Ceremony.

Alpha High School is a private alternative high school known for its nontraditional structure and emphasis on student agency. Instead of teachers, students are paired with "guides," mentors who help them shape individualized learning paths and project portfolios. Core skills are reinforced through two hours of daily app-based AI tutoring, which adapts to each student's pace and proficiency. Classrooms resemble collaborative studios more than lecture halls, and the curriculum often blurs the line between academics and activism, technology and tradition.

Junie thrived in this environment. Her natural curiosity and fierce sense of responsibility made her both a leader among peers and a quiet innovator within the school. Her projects explored intersections of biology and ethics, soil ecology, and social justice, earning praise from Alpha guides and external mentors in the wider community. She was the kind of student who didn't merely complete assignments, she elevated them, turning inquiry into action. While she didn't chase perfection, she earned respect. Her portfolio stood out for its depth, clarity, and purpose. That quiet purpose carried her all the way to the front of the graduation line.

Inside the Performing Arts Center, near the east wing dressing rooms, Junie stands before a mirror adjusting her crimson gown. The fabric is heavy while remaining smooth, cut just right to fall clean over her frame. A white stole rests over her shoulders, edged in silver thread. Her hair is pinned with quiet elegance, just enough curl to frame her face without distracting from her eyes, which are focused, bright, and unmistakably determined.

She isn't valedictorian. That honor went to her friend Anika, a math prodigy with a GPA that has never dipped below perfect. Junie is salutatorian, second in rank but never in presence. Her speech will come first. Somehow, the auditorium is already buzzing about it.

The Performing Arts Center is familiar to most Austinites. Parents whisper that it still smells like new varnish and theater paint. Rows of cushioned seats curve gently around the stage, which is now set with white ferns, school banners, and a single podium under soft lights. Somewhere near the center of the hall, Sonia and Andrew sit holding hands, proud in a way that presses quiet tears to the corners of their eyes.

Backstage, Junie straightens her gown once more, then breathes deeply. She steps into line with the other graduates, her tassel swinging forward over the school crest embroidered on her stole.

It's a good day to stand in front of the world and say something that matters.

The call to line up has just come through the stage manager's headset, and Junie joins the procession with her classmates. The energy backstage is electric. There's nervous laughter, whispered jokes, and the subtle tap of shoes adjusting in place. Junie's heart is fluttering against her ribs. It's the weight of farewell, the thrill of standing on the edge of everything that comes next.

As the line moves, she trails her fingers along the wall, grounding herself in the moment. The scent of hairspray and fresh bouquets mingles with the distant echo of yelling as audience members see their kids, excited to share this moment with them. Her eyes sting from the knowledge that this is the last time they'll be together like this, walking a path they've built side by side.

They file out into the arena of chairs, each step crisp and choreographed. Junie's gaze scans the rows of faces; all angled toward the future. She's excited. Grateful. A little overwhelmed. More than anything, she's ready.

The moment slips by in a heartbeat. The principal's voice cuts through the hum of the auditorium: "Please welcome our salutatorian, Juniper Turbin."

Junie freezes for a fraction of a second. Her name sounds distant, like it was called in a dream. Her palms are damp despite every run-through with her mom and every deep breath she practiced backstage. She brushes her fingers over the hem of her gown one more time, a small anchor to the present.

Her guide gives her a reassuring nod. The line parts slightly, and Junie steps out into the light.

The walk to the stage feels both endless and impossibly fast. Her heels echo in the wide hallway as she makes her way past families craning for photos and underclassmen whispering excitedly. She rounds the last corner and catches a glimpse of the stage, bright under the overheads, then steps behind the final curtain where the stage manager cues her forward.

As she walks toward the podium, applause rises and falls like a soft wave. She keeps her stride steady, but her stomach churns in rhythm with her heartbeat. A mix of stage fright and the gravity of the moment. The awareness that these moments matter and that she's carrying more than her own voice.

At once, she's there. The lights are hot and blinding, the audience a blur of colors and shifting outlines. Somewhere out there, she knows her parents are leaning in with pride.

She finds the microphone, centers herself, and exhales quietly.

"Good morning," she says, her voice clear. "I want to start by thanking the people who built the scaffolding beneath our dreams. Our guides. Our families. Our classmates. And for me, that foundation started at home. I was raised by a teacher and a doctor, though that's not exactly how they describe themselves anymore. Somewhere along the way, they became something else. Scientists, yes, but also stewards of the future. I've watched them every day, quietly, as they taught and healed, questioned and offered care."

She pauses, scanning the crowd until she finds them. She spots her parents, side by side, faces bright with pride. They're not alone in their row. Meera and Theo sit with them, shoulder to shoulder, eyes fixed on her like family. Meera had flown in quietly two days ago, saying the work could wait. "Some moments," she'd told Sonia, "belong to family, whether by blood or by choice."

She exhales through the pause, marking the moment in her mind. Marking the weight of what it means to be seen by loved ones and the very people who shaped her values and courage.

"They never told me to chase greatness," she says at last. "They showed me how to achieve it."

The crowd quiets as she continues. "I grew up watching soil samples instead of cartoons, hearing dinner-table talk about microbial signals and restoration trials. I saw what it looks like when people devote their lives to something that may never bear their names. They taught me that real discovery isn't about claiming ownership; it's about giving something back."

She glances down at her notes, then back to the crowd. "Many of you know I've had my share of hospital days. I learned early that the body can fail you, and sometimes, science doesn't have the answers fast enough. But I also learned that curiosity and compassion can keep you alive in ways medicine can't measure. Every new study, every question my parents asked about how life continues, reminded me that what seems broken can still sustain growth."

A few heads in the audience nod; her classmates adjust and sit taller.

"So, when I think about the work that shaped my family, it isn't just about burial or biology. It's about continuity. About the ways we leave emotional and invisible traces of ourselves, and how those traces build the world after us. The research my parents helped lead taught me that even in decay, there's design. The Earth reuses everything. It's the most generous recycler we know."

She smiles faintly, her confidence growing. "And that lesson belongs to all of us. The future you build, whether in medicine, art, law, or teaching, will depend on how well you listen to what already exists. The world doesn't need us to start from scratch. It needs us to continue what's been started with care."

She smiles brightly before continuing. "So, if we are to build anything lasting, let it be this: a culture where learning is not a ladder, but a language. Where caring isn't a footnote to achievement, but the shape of it. Where progress is measured not just by invention, but by restoration."

Her gaze sweeps across the stage lights and the rows of faces beneath them. "To my fellow graduates, I hope we keep listening to mentors, to strangers, and to each other. When the world hands us a microphone, I hope we speak with clarity and care."

She hesitates, emotion tightening in her throat. "Because that's the part they don't always tell you. It's not enough to know. You have to feel what matters. You have to carry it forward."

Then, with a smile that holds both gratitude and resolve, she nods once, signaling her final line.

"Thank you, and congratulations to the Class of 2037."

Later that afternoon, the Turbins' backyard hums with laughter, music, and the scent of grilled vegetables and spiced lentils. String lights zigzag over the patio as paper lanterns sway gently in the warm June breeze. A banner across the fence reads, "Way to Go, Junie!"

Meera and Theo are among the first guests to arrive. Meera brings a package beautifully wrapped in recycled paper and hand-stamped, and Theo carries a small planter of native wildflowers, the color mix he insists Junie will love.

Junie is radiant in a cotton sundress, her hair pulled up casually, still glowing from the ceremony. She throws her arms around Meera and Theo with barely contained joy.

"I'm so glad you're here," she says, blinking against tears she didn't expect.

"Wouldn't have missed it," Theo replies, already piling a plate with samosas.

"Not for the world," Meera adds, setting the gift on the table and pulling Junie into a quieter hug.

In the corner of the yard, Sonia and Andrew are pouring iced chai and elderflower sodas as neighbors and classmates arrive. The music is lively and plays at a comfortable volume. There's enough space to talk and enough light to laugh.

Junie takes a breath and looks around the space that raised her.

She stands in the middle of this celebration, a gathering of past and future.

The scene remains active as guests arrive and mingle. Junie keeps herself busy, helping her parents create food and drink stations that invite conversation. While she helps carry a tray of mango lassi glasses to the patio, Junie pauses to hear Meera and Sonia chatting at the edge of the lawn.

"Hart Island's been in bloom for three springs straight," Meera says. "You can't walk a path there without seeing native pollinators or field cameras tracking species we haven't seen in a decade. Monarchs, honeybees, and even a family of pectoral sandpipers have been spotted regularly. Wildflowers reseeded themselves along the old burial grounds. It's thriving."

She lifts her glass of chai slightly, as if to toast the thought. "And the soil cores remain clean. Still regenerating. Microbial diversity is stable, and there's even preliminary evidence of atmospheric carbon drawdown in the upper layers. The place has become a benchmark for what legacy restoration can look like when done right."

She pauses, setting the glass down. "But it's not just the soil anymore. We're finally starting to see patterns in nearby populations. The schools adjacent to the restoration zones show steady improvement in respiratory health and immune markers. The same neighborhoods that once registered the highest asthma rates now show the lowest within their districts."

Sonia looks up, interest sharpening. "And the neurodevelopmental data?"

Meera smiles faintly. "That's the part that's still unfolding. We can't make causal claims yet, but early indicators are promising. Infants born in high-exposure regions near active legacy restoration zones are showing slightly higher microbial diversity in their gut biomes by age one. The longitudinal studies suggest that those kids are trending toward stronger immune regulation and even modest improvements in attention span and cognitive flexibility."

Theo steps in, clearly on his way to the buffet table. "In other words, the next generation might literally be growing up with better biological memory."

"Exactly," Meera says. "Not only inherited through genes, but also through the living systems we've repaired. It's slow, but measurable. What we used to call environmental health is starting to look more like generational health."

Sonia nods, eyes reflecting both awe and relief. "People initially scoffed at the natural burials with site stewardship and educational access, but it's become the standard in many states. Texas went first, and the rest followed like dominoes."

Theo rejoins the conversation, now with a second plate. "You know," he says, gently nudging Sonia, "it feels like yesterday you were just starting the permitting battle for the Austin Legacy Garden. When's the last time you were there? How's it going?"

Sonia chuckles. "Oh, don't remind me. It took over a year to get through all the environmental assessments and zoning battles, but once we got the green light, everything moved fairly quickly. It's now part of the McKinney Falls State Park. Nestled near the lower falls. There are restoration plots and guided plantings hosted by area schools. It's beautiful."

Holding a drink just behind her, Andrew steps in with a quieter voice. "I think our parents would've loved to see it. Would've loved to know they're part of it. Part of the living system."

Sonia reaches for his hand, and there's a moment of stillness between them. Theo and Meera offer soft nods that hold memory and agreement all at once.

Sonia glances at the lanterns overhead, her smile softening. "It's my mom's birthday next week. We're planning to spend the morning in the garden. Just a quiet walk. Some flowers. Maybe bring tea and sit on the overlook for a bit. She would've liked that."

Andrew nods beside her. "She loved McKinney Falls. Always said the air smelled sweeter there."

"Now she's part of that air," Sonia replies gently.

A reverent silence follows, a shared pause to honor a presence still felt.

Theo smiles, then glances at Meera. "It's funny. What we once feared to propose is now taught in high school earth sciences. I saw a young kid explain nutrient cycling on a podcast last week."

Meera laughs. "We thought it would take a generation. Turns out, everyone just needed a vocabulary."

She scans the crowd for a moment, then lifts her voice slightly. "Junie! Come over here a sec, woman of the hour."

Junie turns from a conversation with one of her classmates and ambles over, eyebrows raised, glass of lemonade in hand. "What's up?"

"Tell them about São Paulo," Meera says. "Your internship. I want to hear how you described it to the university rep."

Junie blushes lightly. "It's not that dramatic," she says, grinning. "I'm spending the summer with the coalition team down there. They've just opened two new test plots at the edge of the Serra da Cantareira, and they're integrating local traditions into the stewardship model. I'm helping document the plant responses in those transitional zones and creating an interactive soil archive for the community science labs."

"Not that dramatic?" Theo scoffs. "It sounds like you're single-handedly designing the next generation of ecological literacy."

Junie shrugs. "I'm just tagging in where I'm needed, but I'm excited. It feels real. Like I'm starting to take what we've talked about and shape it with my own hands."

Meera raises her glass. "To shaping the world with our own hands."

Everyone clinks in agreement.

A familiar voice cuts across the yard before Junie can drift too far into reflection.

"Junie!"

She turns, instantly recognizing the tall frame of Micah Vasquez, weaving through the crowd on his crutches, sporting a crooked grin.

The same Micah from elementary school and from that hospital room when they were just kids. A year younger, always tagging along, and never quite in her shadow.

They'd grown up together in a kind of orbit around science fairs, school field trips, late-night texts during pandemic lockdowns, and mutual teasing about who really won their spelling bee all those years ago.

Now, he's taller than she remembered, with a confident ease that comes from his own battles. Junie's face lights up.

"Micah! Get over here."

He hands her a gift bag. "You didn't think I'd miss your big day, did you? Salutatorian and São Paulo? That's two international headlines."

She laughs, bumping his shoulder as they walk toward the garden edge. "They'll bury the story under football scores and prom selfies."

"Still," he says, quieter now. "You deserve it. I remember the science fair and how you stayed behind after everyone left just to help me rebuild my project board after it collapsed. You were the one who made me laugh even when I wanted to quit."

Junie's smile softens. "And you were the one who steadied me in my junior year when I was unraveling over my performance at Destination Imagination. You didn't try to fix it. You just stood beside me until I could breathe again. You've always had this clarity. Like you already knew what mattered."

They pause beneath a jacaranda tree, petals scattered like confetti across the lawn.

"How's your summer shaping up?" she asks.

"I'm doing the city fellowship," he says. "Interning with urban planning. They're starting a new green corridor project, and I get to work on the equity mapping team."

Junie's eyes widen. "That's amazing. Micah, that's seriously important."

He shrugs with a mock flourish. "You're not the only one who wants to shape the world."

They pause for a moment, surrounded by friends, voices, and light, with old memories quietly woven into everything around them.

Then Micah nods toward the gift bag still resting in Junie's hands. "You haven't opened your gift."

She blinks, caught off guard. "Oh—right." She tugs gently at the ribbon, opening the bag with care. Inside, nestled in soft tissue, sits a small brass globe, no larger than an apple, polished to a gentle shine.

Junie traces the etched lines of continents with her thumb. "It's beautiful."

Micah smiles. "It's so you can always find your way home. Wherever the world takes you."

She looks up at him, her eyes reflecting the string lights overhead. "That's the best kind of map."

He grins. "Just remember, you don't have to go far to change it."

For a moment, neither of them spoke. The laughter and music around them softens into background light. Then Junie closes her fingers around the globe, holding it, forcing it to remember the tenderness of this night.

Later that evening, as the sun dips behind the rooftops and the lanterns take on their full glow, Junie slips away from the crowd and settles onto the porch steps. Her shoes are off, her plate abandoned, and a crumpled napkin rests between her fingers like a worry stone. The buzz of the gathering hums gently behind her.

Theo notices first. He sidesteps the dessert line and joins her with two sparkling lemonades in hand. "For the newly crowned," he says, handing her one.

"I wasn't crowned," she replies with a soft laugh. "Just recognized, I guess."

"Same thing," he says, easing down beside her. "I've known Nobel winners who weren't recognized half as well."

A pause stretches between them. The kind filled with memory.

Theo glances over at her. "You're thinking about what comes next."

Junie shrugs. "A little. College, obviously. But more than that. The work. The real work. I don't want to just research anymore. I want to implement. Translate what we've learned into something that reaches people who weren't in that auditorium."

"Then that's what you'll do," Theo says simply. "You're ready."

Meera appears a moment later, barefoot and carrying a small notebook. "Hope I'm not interrupting."

"You are," Theo deadpans. "But we'll allow it."

She settles next to Junie on the other side. "I brought you this," she says, handing over the notebook. "It's mostly empty, but I added a few quotes in the margins. People I think you'll like. It's for whatever you need next. Thoughts. Lists. Theories. Confessions."

Junie flips through the pages, pausing at the first quote.

"To care for the earth is to care for its memory."

Meera nods toward the quote. "One of yours, I think."

Junie sets the notebook on her lap, visibly moved.

Laughter erupts from the patio behind them. Sonia is sharing a story from Theo's early lab days, and Andrew is correcting every detail with theatrical flair. There's no need to join them just yet. The future can wait five more minutes.

Junie leans her head against Meera's shoulder. "I think I just want to sit here a little longer."

"Then sit," Meera says, her voice barely above the wind.

And they do.

CHAPTER 26
INHERITANCE

The marker squeaks softly as Sonia draws a row of small rectangles across the whiteboard, each one neatly labeled with a fraction. Behind her, twenty students lean forward, tracking each line as it appears. Some squint in concentration. Others whisper guesses to their table partners. Sonia has been back in the classroom and coaching other teachers for nearly nine years now. She didn't expect to return, and it definitely wasn't something she applied for. But when the principal called, he didn't present it as a job offer. He called it a restoration.

Since her return, the school feels familiar in all the right ways. The hallways are a little brighter, the class sizes a little smaller, and the energy remains with curiosity humming in every corner, students bubbling with questions before she even finishes writing on the board. The classrooms buzz with that same mix of eagerness and mischief, and the playground still erupts each afternoon in a joyful roar that makes her smile every time she hears it.

Sonia sets the marker down and steps back from the board.

"Alright, class. Eyes up here." She taps the row of rectangles; a simple bar model divided into equal parts. "Here's our problem: I baked a pan of brownies and cut it into eight equal pieces. If my brother eats three pieces before dinner, how much of the pan is left? And"—she smiles as a ripple of excitement moves across the room—"who can show that as both a fraction and a picture?"

A hand shoots up. Ava. Always Ava.

"It's five-eighths!" she says, half-standing in her chair. "Because eight pieces total, minus the three he ate, leaves five!"

Sonia nods, warmth spreading through her chest. "Exactly right. Now, I want everyone to show me that on your bar models."

As the students work through their own bar models, Sonia moves between the desks, crouching beside a few who need a nudge and challenging the ones who finish early with a follow-up question. The room hums with quiet concentration, pencils tapping, erasers brushing against paper. When the timer on her desk chimes, groans rise from every corner.

"Alright, mathematicians," she says, clapping her hands once. "Let's wrap it up. Make sure your names are on your papers and stack them on the side table on your way out."

Chairs scrape. Backpacks zip. A few students linger to show her their drawings—a brownie pan sketched with impressive precision, another with pieces shaded in comic-book style. Sonia laughs softly and sends each one out the door with a word of praise. By the time the last clusters of chatter drift into the hallway, the room is settling back into stillness.

Sonia gathers her books and heads for the door. A student lingers by the doorway, waiting for her. He's quiet and thoughtful. He reminds her of Micah.

"Mrs. Turbin?" he says.

"Yes, Tony?" she offers.

"When we round numbers, we lose some detail, but the value stays close, right? So, when we forget things, is it like rounding? It's not gone, just simpler?"

She smiles. "That's an interesting way to see it. We should explore that in math club?"

Tony seems pleased with her answer and smiles as he walks out.

Sonia breathes in, then out.

Some things are worth returning to.

Half a world away, the rhythm is different.

In Pune, the monsoon has ended. The sky is streaked with clouds, and the air is filled with the scent of petrichor. Meera walks along the edge of the sacred grove near Bhira, accompanied by two community health workers and a field biologist from her team. The health workers are there to observe Meera's soil assessments and how local families have responded to reintroducing traditional burial practices. Their presence is part of a broader effort to study the relationship between microbiome recovery and community health. The goal isn't to prove a direct cause, but to trace how renewal in the soil mirrors renewal in the body. How the return of living matter might quietly echo in the lives built above it.

One carries a handheld air sampler, while the other records vital signs of local children interviewed the day before. Meanwhile, the field biologist walks with her eyes focused on the forest floor, spotting early signs of soil regeneration and fungal growth. She's responsible for collecting spore samples and mapping biodiversity blooms across the transition zones, comparing them with control plots outside the grove. Every patch of moss and lichen could indicate microbial activity at work. Their boots sink slightly into the damp soil, and periodically, a root reaches upward like a gentle reminder.

Meera pauses beside a neem tree, its trunk thick with age, its leaves still dripping from yesterday's storm. The burial forest breathes with a quiet density, damp air infused with the sharp scent of leaf mold and the faint musk of fungal bloom. Beneath the canopy, light filters through in fractured green shards, casting slow-moving patterns on the soil. The trees stand close here, their trunks gnarled with age, bark veined with lichen and moss. Somewhere deeper in, a koel calls, echoing like memory through the undergrowth. The ground is soft underfoot, alive with decomposition and rebirth. Mycelium threads lace the roots, visible if you kneel and look closely, whispering stories in a language older than words. The burial forest remains still. Quietly listening. Waiting.

Ritual has been reintroduced quietly here. No grand declarations. Families choosing cloth over plastic, soil over stone. Small things. Old things.

She crouches and presses her palm against the ground.

"They used to say the trees remember," she murmurs. "That roots carry stories. Maybe they do. Maybe they always have."

Behind her, the field biologist calls out. "New bloom. Same plot. Same coordinates as the degradation case."

She slowly stands, wiping her hand on her scarf, and heads to the test site. A modest clearing with a patch of earth that has resisted growth for the past two years now blooms with mycelium. White threads spread outward like script on vellum.

Meera kneels beside it and takes a sample. Her breath is steady. Her hands do not shake.

This, too, is signal.

The persistent presence of scaffolded microbial inheritance is no longer just a theory; it's a monitored, repeatable pattern. Everywhere there's activity, from Pune to São Paulo to Tennessee, the coalition continues to observe its development. Each bloom area is equipped with aerobiological sensors, soil genomic samplers, and seasonal mycoarrays. The fungal networks spreading underground mirror the same scaffolded architectures first seen in Bhira, now layered with microbial and genetic markers that recur across different continents.

The transmission does not follow a linear path. It is fungal and aerosolized. Spores and gene fragments circulate upward, caught in soil exhalation and drawn into local microbial networks. It's what Meera once called "the breath beneath the breath." In these zones, genetic attenuation slows down, sometimes even reversing in microbursts. Children born near them exhibit stronger neuroplasticity, more efficient immune memory, and unexpected mnemonic resilience, with early indicators suggesting fewer developmental delays than nearby control groups.

Everything works together in harmony. The fungal spreads through the grave moss and rootlets, the soil's own gene-sharing metabolism. The fine mist of particulates, once invisible, is now understood as a carrier of dormant signals. The network holds across continents, with parallel results emerging from every test site. For the first time, the coalition does not need to defend its findings. The earth does it for them.

It is similar to how a forest canopy cools a riverbed it never touches, or how coral reefs protect coastlines through wave attenuation even when they are miles from shore. Influence without contact. Shelter without grasp. In nature, proximity fosters protection. The well-being of one system quietly reinforces another. What exists here makes possible what exists there. The network beneath fosters growth above through diffusion. This is how the earth remembers. With resonance.

In Normandy, the remembering is sacred.

Of all the proposed sites, this one was the most politically charged and the most fragile. The coalition didn't lobby. They only presented the evidence. Soil integrity maps, attenuation curves, scaffold profiles. In the end, it wasn't the data that swayed the decision. It was the weight of history.

Every government involved, every flag that once flew there, agreed unanimously that the site would remain a memorial.

The men and women entombed in the Normandy American Cemetery would be returned to the earth over time, with ceremony and caution. Ten years. That was the consensus. A slow re-integration, plot by plot. Rooting memory while allowing the sacred to breathe again.

A dedicated team, led jointly by French and American soil ecologists, has already begun baseline microbial indexing. No soil will be disturbed without full ancestral tracing, and every transition will include the ritual accompaniment of blessings and song to recognize each moment of life returned to the Earth.

What rests here carries undeniable grief, but it also carries hope for the future.

Even in reverence, the Earth knows what to do with that.

As Normandy starts its respectful journey back to the Earth, other sites keep progressing with their own patterns of change.

In Utrecht, Lotte van Dalen manages the first controlled replication of microbial bloom post-burial reintroduction. Twenty-seven reclaimed plots, previously sealed, have been turned into natural interments with family consent. The results surprise the coalition team. Within two years, fungal biodiversity doubled. Pediatric health indicators in adjacent communities slightly improved. Nothing dramatic, but it was undeniable.

Kaoru Watanabe's team in Japan observes similar patterns. The shizensō communities maintain elevated child health metrics, indicating advanced language skills and strong memory retention beyond expected baselines.

Eduardo in São Paulo films a short video of children planting wild-flowers at the edge of a restored burial site. The ground, once lifeless, now seems to sing.

Not all calls to restoration are answered the same way. The Shepherd's Stand Alliance, once a galvanizing spiritual force behind ethical reburial practices, has waned in influence. What began as a chorus of faith leaders standing in defense of Earth's memory fractured over time. Some branches urged faster reclamation, others retreated entirely as the science deepened.

The Vatican remained quiet far longer than expected. Inquiries were made, and the coalition issued a briefing, discreet and densely footnoted. Then, months later, a message arrived. It was expected that it would come from the Congregation for the Doctrine of the Faith, but instead, it came from the Pope's own ecological advisor. It was short and simple.

"Life given back to the soil is not lost. It is entrusted."

They took it as a blessing.

Since then, a few dioceses have started pilot programs to include natural burials alongside traditional rites by reading from Genesis and offering mycelial pairings. The sacred, it turns out, have always known how to transition into renewal.

With global soil studies maturing and spiritual debates settling into new forms of ritual, attention returns insistently to the children. The first children studied in the attenuation zones are turning fifteen.

Zoe Sanders, one of Andrew's earliest flagged cases, now attends a charter school with an emphasis on kinetic learning. Her delays have stabilized. She doesn't read as fluently as some of her peers, but she builds models from scratch using cardboard and equations only she under-stands. Her teachers describe her as "spatially brilliant."

Mateo Cruz, who didn't respond to his name for nearly a year, now plays piano by ear. He can't explain how he knows where the notes go; he just does. His EEGs still show anomalies, but the patterns have shifted. Less stutter. More song.

Dell Children's Medical Center remains an important contributor to the research. Dell Children's, where a father's inquiry led to connections and inspiration that have rippled across continents and generations. In a back corner, beyond the new EEG suite, a quiet memorial wall has been added to the pediatric neurology wing.

Andrew didn't ask for it. Someone on the team suggested it after a staff meeting. Within a month, it was real. A photo wall of trees. Roots. Soil. Each frame is labeled with a patient ID and a single word. "Remembered."

One evening, after rounds, Andrew walks past it alone.

He stops at a photo of a cypress tree. Beneath it, the word: Kaylen.

He takes a few moments to reflect and remember.

The story isn't ending, but the pace of it has changed. The coalition meets less frequently now. Governments have begun to shoulder what was once theirs alone. Local jurisdictions now fund rewilding plots, the integration of natural burial education into public health curricula, and the building of local task forces to manage soil monitoring. The baton has been passed, hand to hand, nation to nation.

The coalition members meet in person for the first time in over a year.

Not in a lab or a conference room.

In a field.

A rural research center in the Upper Cumberland region of eastern Tennessee offers its land for the next study phase. Nestled just outside Cookeville, near the edge of Standing Stone State Forest, the center provides forty acres of unsealed hardwood forest. The location, once part of an experimental agriculture and soil resilience project, now serves as a model transition site. Controlled burial zones. Full-spectrum biodiversity monitoring. Maternal health tracking in surrounding communities. Partnerships with nearby schools and clinics. Here, restoration is the curriculum, clinic, and canopy.

Theo brings his laptop and three flasks of something he calls coffee. Meera brings local soil samples in hand-labeled jars. Kaoru brings his silence. Eduardo brings a photo of the São Paulo bloom wall. Lotte brings her boots.

Andrew and Sonia bring hope and vision.

They walk the perimeter purposefully, noting early signs of growth. Fungi near the elder grove. Worm paths in compost beds. The wind moves differently here. It seems quieter. It feels awake.

As the sun dips low, Meera stands near the central clearing and reads from her notes.

"We are here to study the soil and to learn," she says. "We are here to see if the past wants to teach us something."

The wind answers.

That night, they stay in the bunkhouse near the edge of the forest. Sonia curls up with her book on the couch. Andrew stands by the porch, watching fireflies rise like scattered signals.

Theo steps beside him, nursing the last of his "coffee."

"We did a thing," Theo says.

"We did," Andrew agrees.

"Think the world will notice?"

"Maybe not right away."

Theo nods. "That's okay. Soil takes time."

Behind them, a light blinks on. Meera steps onto the porch, arms folded against the cool.

"You know," she says, "in some traditions, they say silence is the first form of memory."

Andrew smiles.

"Then maybe this," he gestures to the dark, the stars, the quiet earth, "is the loudest remembering we've ever done."

They stand in the silence together.

Letting the Earth speak.

Listening back.

A LETTER FROM THE AUTHOR

If you've made it this far, thank you. You've walked with these characters through mystery, doubt, discovery, and decision. You've entertained the possibility that what we think we know about the body, about the Earth, and about each other might not be complete.

I first came up with the idea for *Drift* in the mid-1990s. It sat undeveloped for far too long. I'm writing this story now because I have questions about the world we live in and how we influence it. I hope you ask your own questions too.

Much of our world operates under the illusion of certainty. We build our systems, our science, even our relationships on frameworks we trust to be complete. What if we can't see the whole picture? What if nature, quietly and steadily, has been trying to tell us that the code we trust is only part of that picture?

When I'm outside biking over trails in Colorado, listening to the rustle of aspen trees, or sitting beside a campfire enjoying the sound of the wind, it feels like the earth is speaking. Quietly. You have to listen and observe nature to hear it truly. Nature doesn't always offer direct answers; it offers patterns, rhythms, and quiet feedback. You have to slow down to catch them and look for the signs. You must be present to learn.

My dad once told me that you can't ask for evidence of God. Instead, you have to be sharp enough to recognize the signs that God is present.

The spirit of curiosity runs throughout this book. The science here is fictional, yes, but it's rooted in real patterns. Genetic drift, ecosystem dependence, cultural memory, and the way life evolves without asking for our permission. I hope this story sparks your curiosity, just as the rustling of trees or the changing of seasons always sparks mine.

Stay open. Stay grounded. Ask the right questions.

I don't pretend to have it all figured out. However, I firmly believe in listening to nature and to one another. That's where discovery begins.

Wayne

ACKNOWLEDGMENTS

This book would not exist without the support, insight, and generosity of many people who walked with me through its creation.

To my partner, Peter Zeihan, thank you for encouraging every creative leap, for believing in this story long before it had a name, and for giving me the space to pursue it fully. Your support continues to widen the horizon of what I imagine possible.

To my niece, Lorain Amrocio, whose guidance, expertise, and steady coaching shaped both the storytelling and the confidence behind it. You gave your time freely and pushed me to see what the manuscript could become. I am deeply grateful.

To Benjamin Sledge, who brought the visual identity of this project to life. Your cover work and design instinct gave the story a face before it found its readers. Your art can be explored at benjaminsledge.com, and I am honored to feature your talent here.

To everyone who offered encouragement, critique, or simple curiosity along the way, thank you for helping me carry this book to completion.